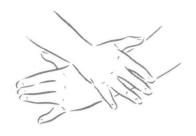

THE ESSENTIALS OF

McTIMONEY
CHIROPRACTIC

Elizabeth Andrews and Anthea Courtenay

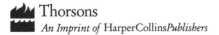

Thorsons
An Imprint of HarperCollins*Publishers*

Thorsons

An Imprint of HarperCollins*Publishers*

77–85 Fulham Palace Road,

Hammersmith, London W6 8JB

Published by Thorsons 1999

10 9 8 7 6 5 4 3 2 1

A catalogue record for this book
is available from the British Library

ISBN 0 7225 3747 6

Text illustrations by Peter Cox Associates

Printed and bound in Great Britain by
Woolnough Bookbinding Ltd, Irthlingborough, Northamptonshire

CONTENTS

ACKNOWLEDGEMENTS

The authors would like to thank the many chiropractors, doctors and patients who have contributed their knowledge and experience to this book. Particular thanks are owing to Dawn Acres, Jillian Baldwin, Madeleine Brzeski, Dr David Buckler, Susan Cartlidge, Lynda Clark, Margie Craib, Dr Christina Cunliffe, Valerie Duvall, Tony Gilmore, Dana Green, Stanley Harding, Bronwen Herbertson, Shelagh James-Hudson, Fiona Macrae, The McTimoney Chiropractic Association, Ian Miller, Ian Pearson, Caroline Ritherden, Daphne Tomlin, Dr Phil Whitaker and Mark Windsor.

INTRODUCTION

The inspiration and spirit of one man, John McTimoney,
has spread across the world – not only in the form of
hundreds of practitioners who feel privileged to know
and understand his methods but also in the thousands
and thousands of grateful patients.

This book looks at all the principal features of
McTimoney chiropractic, beginning with its history
and showing how the technique fits in with the more
mainstream chiropractic scene. What to expect in a
treatment session is described fully and clearly, together
with all the many other types of problems the technique
can help, backed up by many case histories – some
extraordinary.

A Widespread Answer to a Prevalent Problem

Manipulating the spine is one of the oldest and most widespread therapies in the world, going back to 2700 BC. Today both osteopathy and chiropractic are becoming increasingly accepted by medical doctors, and chiropractic is the most widely recognized complementary or alternative therapy throughout the world.

Despite this, the figures published by the UK's National Back Pain Association make alarming reading. The highest incidences occur in the nursing, construction, agriculture and retail food and water industries. This costs these industries billions, and the health care system hundreds of millions, every year.

Back injury is the largest single cause of long-term sick leave, with 60 per cent of adults suffering back problems annually. About one-third of these become chronic sufferers. The problem is not only to do with advancing years; alarmingly, there is an increased prevalence among 16- to 24-year-olds, and there are no regulations to protect children who have to carry heavy satchels of books to and from school.

Common causes of back problems across the professions are found in poor workplace design and inadequate or infrequent training for both manual and sedentary workers. Problems also occur from extended working in fixed body positions, and are compounded by poor car seating and bad driving posture. Professional drivers – bus, lorry and taxi drivers – are especially likely to suffer.

The Essentials of McTimoney Chiropractic

Lifestyle factors also contribute to the problem. While the highest incidences are found in *all* sedentary and *all* manual work, lowest incidence is found when tasks and activities are varied. Lack of exercise, poorly supportive or sagging mattresses and sofas or chairs, and long periods of slouching in front of the television are common causes.

While only between 1 and 2 per cent of back investigations result in surgery, 85 per cent receive no differential diagnosis at all.

Common diagnoses include non-specific low back pain (which includes ligamentous strain, joint dysfunction, disc protrusion or prolapse, with or without nerve root compression), facet joint pain, sacro-iliac joint dysfunction, degenerative disc or joint disease and osteoporosis. Common effects of these are loss of the ability to walk, sit, bend or lift, incontinence, intractable pain, sciatic pain, or loss of sensation or numbness in the limbs and feet. As with any lengthy period of ill health, especially when accompanied by pain, there is frequently also tiredness and depression.

These facts show that there is plenty of scope for an aspiring chiropractor. Yet chronic back pain is only one of the many problems that chiropractic can help. This book outlines the kind of help a McTimoney chiropractor can offer, whether the problem is acute or chronic, and includes details of the importance of the practitioner's taking a good initial history, carrying out the treatment, and advising patients and their families on preventative measures and how to help themselves.

Chapter 8 describes how the technique has been developed as a properly validated treatment for animals. An experienced animal practitioner, Dana Green, says 'When I go to a stable, I sometimes treat everything that moves – horses, dogs, riders, grooms, the lot!'

A Philosophy for Health

Perhaps the words of experienced McTimoney chiropractor Jo Hanstead best illustrates the spirit of McTimoney chiropractic:

A colleague and I recently gave a lecture/demonstration on McTimoney chiropractic to 60 doctors. The majority responded with interest and the usual surprise at the gentleness and effectiveness of the technique. Question time was an opportunity for the more sceptical members to express their views. An orthopaedic surgeon, who himself carried out manipulation under general anaesthetic, stated that he found that far more force was needed to move bones than we appeared to be putting in. We responded that this was his experience – and that our experience was that very little force was needed to make adjustments. Looking back, I think he put his finger on just what it is that we offer that is so unique, but also hard to understand and believe by those with a conventional background. Our basic philosophy is no different from that taught to other chiropractors. Our practitioners have their own philosophies and beliefs which are as diversified and as individual as they are. The technique is a set of many types of adjustment which require a level of sensitivity and dexterity to perform, and which can be learned with practice.

We learn from our own experience that the results of the treatment are undeniably impressive. Chronic and acute conditions consistently respond in ways that are nothing less than remarkable. And we don't move bones! As it is extolled to our students, we supply a packet of kinetic energy – the body's Innate Intelligence makes the best use of it for that person at that time.

We continually have the philosophy reinforced by our own experience, not beliefs, that we do not force realignment, we merely initiate change. Our patients' responses teach us day by day a simple awe of the power of Innate Intelligence. We are no more noble or altruistic than any others in the healing arts, but our trust in the technique becomes a rock, the strength of which is felt by our patients and is reflected in our work.

Practical training is by direct transmission from generation to generation in a direct line from John McTimoney. Being a living technique, each generation of teachers hones the technique, guided by peer consensus. Students are gently led by experienced practitioners towards their own understanding of, and trust in the technique.

This book will inspire anyone interested in studying a gentle, non-invasive yet brilliantly effective technique. It also gives details of the type of personality and study required to become an expert practitioner. Potential patients, be they back pain sufferers or in pain for other reasons, will welcome not only the gentleness of the technique but also the advice on how to help themselves to prevent a recurrence of their symptoms.

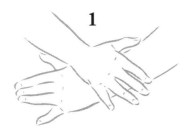

THE BIRTH OF CHIROPRACTIC

I have answered the time-worn question – what is life?

D D PALMER

Spinal manipulation is an ancient art. The earliest written account of it has been found in a Chinese document, the *Kong Fou*, dated around 2700 BC; manipulative therapies were practised throughout the civilizations of the ancient world. The early fathers of medicine, the Greek physicians Hippocrates and Galen, practised spinal manipulation and preached the importance of the spine in relation to health. As well as using manual adjustment, Hippocrates is credited with inventing a mechanical device for stretching the spine by traction; he also recommended sitting on patients if necessary!

As time went on, much of this early wisdom was lost with the destruction of hundreds of libraries after the fall of

Rome in AD 476. In a Europe where health was constantly endangered by plagues, physicians were hesitant to lay their hands on patients. Manipulative techniques continued among country people by naturally gifted bonesetters. Thus the scene was set for the divide between orthodox medicine and chiropractic, which, along with osteopathy, came to be regarded as an 'alternative' therapy. Both these techniques were met with distrust and disbelief by the medical establishment.[1]

Today chiropractic is the most widely recognized alternative (or complementary) therapy throughout the world. In the US, chiropractors have something of the status of family doctors. In the UK, both mainstream and McTimoney chiropractic are taught as recognized degree courses. This very recent recognition has arrived after a long, hard struggle, ironically rendered the harder by the enthusiasm and individuality of its pioneers.

Daniel David Palmer

The history of chiropractic began in 1895 when Harvey Lillard walked into the office of Daniel David Palmer, a practitioner of 'magnetic healing' living in Davenport, Iowa. This method of healing involved the laying on of hands. Palmer was a short, thickset 50-year-old, his mane of greying hair and heavy beard enhancing his compelling personality. As Palmer began questioning Lillard about his condition, Lillard explained that 17 years before he had been stooping when he felt something give in his back; almost immediately, he'd lost his hearing.

Palmer tried giving Lillard magnetic treatment, to no avail. On examining Lillard, he found a painful and prominent vertebra in his upper spine. Yes, said Lillard, that was the place that had hurt when he'd lost his hearing. Palmer asked him to lie face down on the treatment table, and exerted an energetic manual thrust on the vertebra in question. Shortly afterwards, Lillard announced that he was beginning to hear again. The first chiropractic adjustment had been made.

Palmer later wrote that the event was no accident; the adjustment 'was accomplished with an object in view, and the result expected was obtained. There was nothing crude about this adjustment; it was specific.' He had in fact been working towards this for some years.

Palmer had learned the skill of magnetic healing from Paul Caster, an internationally known practitioner, and had been practising it for some 10 years when he encountered his patient Harvey Lillard. Magnetic healing (which derived from the 'magnetism' developed by the 18th-century Austrian healer Franz Mesmer) was just one form of unconventional therapy enjoying popularity in the US at the time. Medicine, particularly in the West and Midwest, was far from satisfactory. There were few doctors, and many of these were poorly trained. Medical treatment consisted of purges, blood-letting and a heavy-handed use of such drugs as were available. There was also a lively non-medical trade in spurious elixirs based largely on alcohol.

On the East coast, medicine was progressing towards its present scientific basis, as it was in Europe. In France, Pasteur had established his theory of germs in the 1860s, while in England, Joseph Lister was working obsessively on establishing the case for antiseptic surgery. However, in the US the sheer lack of trained doctors in rural areas had encouraged throughout the 19th century a general interest in natural healing methods: these included diet, herbs, exercise, electricity, purges, bone-setting, religious healing, magnetic healing, sunshine therapy, homoeopathy and mineral baths. This setting provided a fertile seedbed for the growth of two new major schools: osteopathy and chiropractic.

Osteopathy came first. In 1864 the three children of a country doctor, Andrew Taylor Still, died of spinal meningitis, a tragedy crystallizing Still's disillusionment with orthodox medicine. The son of a Methodist preacher and healer, Still had studied engineering and trained briefly in medicine. The two studies conjoined when he developed the theory that many ailments stem from distortions or malfunctions in the structure of the body.

Still's theory was that the body cannot function properly unless it is structurally sound: if a faulty structure is rectified, the body's own 'life-force' will take over to restore health.

Palmer, meanwhile, was on his own quest for the cause of disease. He, too, had observed the failures of medicine. 'Why drug the entire body,' he was to ask, 'when only one organ is sick?' Although he seems to have had some success as a healer, he felt that this method only addressed the symptoms of disease, not its fundamental cause. Like Still – and many others before him – he believed that the body possessed its own natural healing forces. He wrote later: 'One question was always uppermost in my mind in my search for the Cause of Disease. I desired to know why one person was ailing and his associate working in the same shop at the same bench was not. This question was answered in September, 1895, with my first chiropractic adjustment.' If the vertebrae of the spine were misaligned, he reasoned, this must affect the nervous system; adjust the spine and healing will follow.

With a regular clientele visiting him for magnetic healing, he had ample opportunity to test his theories. Shortly after his first adjustment, he was visited by a patient whose heart trouble was not responding to orthodox medical treatment. Palmer examined his spine and, as he described it later, 'found a displaced vertebra pressing against the nerves which innervate the heart'. He adjusted the vertebra and the patient's condition immediately began to improve. 'Then I began to clearly reason, if two diseases so dissimilar as deafness and heart trouble came from a spinal impingement, causing a pressure upon nerves, were not other diseases due to a similar cause?'

It is understandable that he should come to such a conclusion; it is also curious that Palmer's first two chiropractic cases were of types that today are scarcely obvious candidates for spinal manipulation. But success in an increasing number of cases, together with his observation that displaced vertebrae were the rule in the sick, rather than the exception, seemed to prove Palmer's theory of a basic cause of ill-health.

Among Palmer's patients was the Reverend Samuel Weed, whom Palmer asked to name his new treatment. Did he know of a Greek word for 'done by hand'? Weed came up with *cheiro praktikos*, and from this the word 'chiropractic' was coined.

Palmer knew perfectly well that people had been adjusting vertebrae for the relief of disease for thousands of years. His system, however, was new, as he stressed in no uncertain terms:

I am the originator, the Fountain Head of the essential principle that disease is the result of too much or not enough functionating. I created the art of adjusting vertebrae, using the spinous and transverse processes[2] as levers, and named the mental act of accumulating knowledge, the cumulative function, corresponding to the physical vegetative function – growth of intellectual and physical – together, with the science, art and philosophy – Chiropractic … It was I who combined the science and art and developed the principles thereof. I have answered the time-worn question – what is life!

A Proliferation of Schools

Over the years, D D Palmer and his followers refined and revised his theories and the practice of chiropractic. A specific terminology was introduced: displacements in the spine came to be called 'subluxations'.[3] The concept of the life-force in the individual was interpreted in Palmer terms as 'Innate Intelligence' which was linked to a creative 'Universal Intelligence'. This philosophy, which his followers came to call *Vitalism*, was important to Palmer, and he never failed to stress the moral and religious duties of the chiropractor:

Chiropractic science includes biology – the science of life – in this world, and the recognition of a spiritual existence in the next … Displacement of any part of the skeletal frame

The Essentials of McTimoney Chiropractic

may press against nerves, which are the channels of communication, intensifying or decreasing their carrying capacity, creating either too much or not enough functioning, an aberration known as disease ...

Spinal subluxations (misalignment) could produce a wide range of symptoms – deafness and heart disease, headaches, digestive disorders, skin problems, let alone backache. No need for drugs; no point in treating symptoms; simply find and correct the subluxation, Palmer believed, and healing would take place.

It is not surprising that Palmer incurred the enmity of a medical profession which increasingly viewed disease as visited on patients through external agencies such as germs. Modern, allopathic (drug-based) medicine is based on the premise that disease can be suppressed, while complementary therapies are mainly based on encouraging the patient's own powers of self-healing. The schism between 'Vitalists' and 'Scientists' was later to emerge among Palmer's own followers, although Palmer himself totally rejected the latter approach.

Despite this, his early students (half of whom were women) included medical doctors. His first 15 graduates included five doctors, among them J S Riley, MD, PhD, who wrote in 1925: 'Some of his cures seemed like miracles, and while we had studied medicine, osteopathy, magnetic healing, mental science, etc., we saw chiropractic doing a work that all the others combined could not do.' Chiropractic patients in those days – as is often the case today – tended to be those for whom conventional medical treatment had failed.

By 1897, the Palmer School of Chiropractic was offering a six-month course; it had one student in 1898 and a dozen by 1903. One early student was Willard Carver, a lawyer whose specialization in negligence work had aroused his interest in anatomy and physiology. In the history of chiropractic, Palmer, his son Bartlett Joshua (known as B J), and Carver are known as the 'trinity of giants': D D Palmer was the Founder, B J Palmer the Developer, and Carver titled himself the Constructor. On the side of the 'Scientists', Carver tried to 'prove' chiropractic, and described subluxations (misalignments) as 'abnormal curves of the spine which lead to muscle imbalance.' He made some valuable contributions to the development of chiropractic; he recognized that the 'nerve flow' could be impeded in other parts of the body as well as the spine. He also stressed the importance of correct posture, and made the important observation that if the spine is distorted at one level, the body's attempts to compensate will produce distortions at other levels.

Carver went on to found and run four chiropractic schools; others were also springing up. For his part, D D Palmer founded the Portland College of Chiropractic in partnership with a surgeon and a homoeopath, and in 1907 launched the Palmer-Gregory School of Chiropractic with medical doctor Alva Gregory in Oklahoma City. He also handed over the original and rapidly expanding Davenport, Iowa school to his son B J; as more and more students graduated they also began setting up small schools of their own, often introducing their own ideas and variations.

Opposition

Although the early chiropractic students included a fair sprinkling of osteopaths, chiropractic was to be strongly opposed by osteopathy. Both groups had started mainly with patients who could not afford expensive medical treatment or who lived in districts where doctors were few. By the early 1900s both treatments were well established and were attracting observers and students from overseas. As time went by, osteopaths began to collect a more fashionable clientele, founding medical schools and allying themselves with the orthodox medical profession.

In 1906 D D Palmer was jailed under the Medical Practice Acts, instigated by the medical profession in the 1880s to prohibit non-medical persons from practising medicine without a licence. That same year his ambitious young son B J published a book on chiropractic (he'd written four more by 1910) which D D regarded as anatomically and physiologically erroneous. B J had also given himself the title of Developer of Chiropractic, and granted himself the advanced degree of PhC. D D responded with his own book, *The Science, Art and Philosophy of Chiropractic*; it, too, has been criticized for its anatomical and physiological inaccuracies, although one writer comments that Palmer's writings 'remain remarkable considering that he was self-taught in these sciences'.[4]

By 1910 D D Palmer had also fallen out with Dr Gregory, and the Palmer-Gregory School broke up. In 1911 he returned to Davenport and made a further attempt at working with his son at the Palmer School of Chiropractic; it failed. D D then set up a rival school, the Universal Chiropractic College, two streets away; again, he quarrelled with his partners. He died in Los Angeles in 1913. One account of his death points the finger at the after-effects of an accident occurring during his last visit to Davenport, when he was hit by a car: '[It] was driven by B J, and largely unsubstantiated charges of patricide would linger for years.'⁵

If there is a soap-opera element in the early history of chiropractic, with its larger-than-life characters and history of familial and professional rivalries, this should not blind us to the fact that the focus of all this was a system of healing, of caring for the sick and nurturing the healthy, which was doing a large number of people a great deal of good. It is one of the paradoxes of human creativity that prophets, healers and gurus who have a genuine truth to impart are often afflicted by oversized egos.

B J Palmer

Bartlett Joshua Palmer, born in 1881, was ambitious, domineering, a self-styled genius who could brook no opposition. His interests were not limited to chiropractic; he started the second commercial broadcasting station in the US – all the better for advertising chiropractic, of course.

In 1906 B J and his wife Mabel, who also practised and taught chiropractic, moved to the first of a series of larger premises in the district where the campus of the Palmer College stands today. By 1915 enrolments were over 800; in 1918 there were 1,862 students, drawn from all walks of life and professions, including some medical doctors and osteopaths. By now the curriculum included anatomy, physiology, symptomatology, pathology and diagnosis, toxicology, obstetrics and dissection, as well as the science and philosophy of chiropractic.

Although self-educated like his father, B J worked hard to give the profession a scientific basis. A major contribution was his introduction of X-ray equipment to the school as early as 1909 (marking one major difference between chiropractic and osteopathy, and later, McTimoney Chiropractic). By 1910 the school had collected a library of several hundred glass negatives of the spine which were used for research and teaching. B J also assembled the world's largest osteological museum.

B J believed that if the idea of Innate Intelligence was properly understood, everything else would follow, and that healing worked from 'above down and from inside to out'. His greatest ambition was 'to see the chiropractic principle and practice perpetuate itself in its purity for posterity, unfettered and unshackled by antipodal restrictions, legal or otherwise, so that the greatest number of sick under chiropractic care may get well in the quickest possible time.'

The 'antipodal restrictions' he refers to were the Medical Practice Acts in place between the First and Second World Wars in the United States, under which thousands of chiropractors were prosecuted and imprisoned, often having been 'set up' by agents paid by doctors to impersonate patients. In California in 1921, 450 chiropractors convicted of practising medicine without a licence were given the alternative of paying a fine or going to jail. They all chose jail. The effect was to arouse public sympathy; newspaper

The Birth of Chiropractic

offices were bombarded with letters of protest, not only defending chiropractors but also blaming organized medicine for putting up 'decoy evidence' against them.

In the first half of the 20th century the American medical profession was particularly jealous of its status. Not only were chiropractors claiming cures which were regarded as medical impossibilities, their patients were pleased with their treatment and were paying less for it than doctors were charging. And they were advertising their services in a self-declamatory fashion which must have been particularly annoying. The printing presses of the Davenport school churned out millions of tracts; B J Palmer alone published more than 35 books, and promoted chiropractic as the cure for all ills.

Divisions were also on the increase among chiropractic practitioners themselves. B J Palmer invented a technique, vividly entitled 'Hole In One' (HIO), in which only the first or second cervical vertebra (at the top of the neck) was adjusted. He also created, in collaboration with Dr Dossa D Evins of the Palmer School faculty, a diagnostic tool called a *neurocalometer*, a heat-sensing device whose purpose was to locate areas of temperature differential along the spine. In a talk at the Davenport school entitled 'The Hour has Struck', B J told his audience of thousands that no chiropractor could practise without a neurocalometer, and that any chiropractor not using this with the HIO was incapable of practising honestly. He lost the support of a large number of chiropractors, and his influence began to wane.

There were further divisions in the profession between the 'straights', who believed in practising chiropractic alone, and the 'mixers', who saw value in including other therapies where appropriate, such as naturopathy or homoeopathy. Two main schools developed: the International Chiropractors Association (ICA), founded by the 'straights' in Davenport in 1926, and the National (now American) Chiropractic Association (NCA), founded in 1930 by the 'mixers'. Both the ICA and the NCA referred to doctors those cases that lay beyond their scope of treatment.

Despite the controversies and divisions, chiropractic continued to spread and, by 1931, 39 American states had granted legal recognition to doctors of chiropractic. And although a number of fly-by-night schools continued to come and go, training in the main schools was vastly improved by the introduction of medical doctors on the staff and medical methods of diagnosis.

B J remained active, fascinated by both science and his own theories. In 1935 he produced an instrument for reading brainwaves and their conduction through the spinal cord. In the same year he established a research clinic in the school, where he received the seriously ill; it had a full medical and nursing staff, a diagnostic laboratory and physical medicine section. He also operated a chiropractic facility for mental patients, and continued to preach the importance of Innate Intelligence. By the 1950s he was lecturing on Innate Intelligence and the spiritual significance of sex and phallicism (he had a rare collection of phallic symbols). He died in 1961.

He was Elbert Hubbard, Titus Oates, Baron Munchausen and P T Barnum all rolled into one, yet to his research clinic at midcentury would come "hopeless" and terminal cases –

*some on referral from the Mayo and Cleveland clinics – to
leave apparently cured ... Controversial and colourful, he
outraged his detractors in both medicine and chiropractic as
much with his style as with his propositions, yet provided
an environment for legitimate spinal research and
development.*

Acceptance

Despite its somewhat eccentric beginnings, chiropractic
has become the most widely practised therapy in the
world after medicine and dentistry. Its history almost
everywhere has been one of medical opposition and public
support. It is not only popular with patients, but by now
has been legally recognized by many governments. For
although the early claims that it could cure just about
everything have been largely (though not totally) dropped,
it has been shown to provide a safe, drug-free therapy that
is effective with a wide range of musculo-skeletal
disorders, and often improves other conditions.

Over the last century – and in particular the last 25 years –
chiropractic has grown up. There have been changes in
both theory and practice: techniques have been refined and
new ones introduced; educational standards are constantly
improving, and there is a greater understanding of the
anatomy and function of the nervous system in both
chiropractic and medicine.

In the US chiropractic expanded particularly rapidly after
the Second World War, although prosecutions continued in
some states into the 1960s. Since 1971, chiropractors have
been licensees in all 50 American states as primary health-
care providers, legally recognized as providing an

alternative medical service to general practitioners; in 1972 the US Congress voted to make chiropractic available under Medicare. Today in America there are around 50,000 practising chiropractors treating 15–20 million patients.

Since the inception of the Council on Chiropractic Education (CCE) which is recognized by the US Department of Health, Education, and Welfare as the accrediting body for chiropractic colleges, many of the smaller colleges have disappeared and educational curricula have been standardized. The Doctor of Chiropractic degree has the same standing as a medical degree, and American chiropractors are entitled to call themselves doctors.

The divisions between Vitalists and Scientists, and 'straights' and 'mixers', have survived. Members of the American Chiropractors Association (ACA) regard themselves as holistic physicians rather than spinal specialists. They are 'mixers', incorporating into their treatment other therapies, particularly nutrition and mineral and vitamin supplementation; many of them have been forerunners in this field, as well as in the application of Applied Kinesiology (see page 53). The International Chiropractors Association continues to represent the 'straights'.

A Worldwide Therapy

From its American roots, chiropractic has spread around the world, particularly the English-speaking world, with substantial numbers of practitioners in Canada and

Australia and a respectable number in New Zealand and South Africa. There are also a certain number in the Far and Middle East, and Africa.

In Europe chiropractic has followed an interesting path. Legal and other restrictions have encouraged European chiropractors, particularly in Britain, to become specialists in spinal and joint problems. And, apart from within Britain, chiropractic is much better known than osteopathy throughout Europe.

The European Chiropractors Union (ECU), formed in 1932 as an umbrella group for various national chiropractors' associations, ensures some cohesiveness among its members. The ECU has worked hard to improve educational standards, and more recently to deal with the legal issues arising within the European Community (EC).

Legislation

The law on non-medical therapies varies from country to country in Europe. Under current British law, for example, anyone may set up as a practitioner of anything with no training at all provided the law does not expressly forbid it. At the time of writing this situation is about to change: the 1994 Chiropractic Act comes into force in Britain in 1999, and then only registered practitioners will be allowed to set up as chiropractors.

Chiropractic in Britain

If chiropractic is relatively little known in Britain, this is largely owing to the historical accident which brought more osteopaths to England early in the 20th century, and their speed in setting up osteopathic training schools. The British School of Osteopathy was founded as early as 1917, followed by a number of competing osteopathic colleges, whereas up until 1965 anyone wanting a proper training in chiropractic had to go to the US.

Today, the number of chiropractors continues to increase, with some 900 practising in the UK and four voluntary professional organizations: the British Chiropractic Association (BCA), the British Association of Applied Chiropractic (BAAC), the McTimoney Chiropractic Association (MCA), and the Scottish Chiropractic Association (SCA). The largest and oldest of these, the BCA, was formed in 1925, its aims being 'to handle chiropractic, assist its growth and be prepared for protective measures'.

Perhaps because of its small numbers, chiropractic in Britain has not suffered from the same medical opposition as elsewhere. Yet there have been disputes within the profession itself (B J Palmer's 'Hole in One' aroused controversy in the UK as in the US), and European chiropractors have also been divided into 'straights' and 'mixers'.

Qualifications

In 1965 the Anglo-European College of Chiropractic (AECC) was formed in Bournemouth, offering a four-year full-time course. The standards of the US Council on Chiropractic Education have become accepted worldwide, and there are reciprocal councils in Canada and Australia to accredit colleges in these countries. In 1984 the European Chiropractors' Union established a European

Council on Chiropractic Education (ECCE), a self-governing accrediting body, which accredited Britain's AECC in 1992. The UK's Council for National Academic awards had already validated a BSc degree in chiropractic in 1988; in 1992 this was enhanced to a BSc (Honours) degree after four years, and a post-graduate Diploma in chiropractic after the fifth year, now validated by the University of Portsmouth. Nevertheless, many BCA members practising in Britain today trained in the US or Canada.

McTimoney Practice

In the 1940s, two or three members of the BCA, anxious to pass on their skills, began to teach patients informally on an apprenticeship basis. One of these was Dr Mary Walker, a graduate of the Palmer School, who taught John McTimoney. In the 1950s and sixties McTimoney developed his own techniques for both people and animals – as will be described more fully in Chapter 2. In 1972 he founded the McTimoney Chiropractic School in Oxford, from which today's McTimoney Chiropractic College descends. McTimoney Chiropractors formed the Institute of Pure Chiropractic, now known as the McTimoney Chiropractic Association (MCA). One of McTimoney's graduates in turn, Hugh Corley, founded his own school and formed the British Association of Applied Chiropractic (BAAC).

Clinical Trials

Although the BCA and AECC have always adopted a strongly scientific approach, until recently chiropractic has been regarded in Britain as very much an alternative therapy. A problem which all alternative or complementary therapies suffer from is the medical establishment's attitude of extreme caution – and often disbelief – towards therapies which have not undergone medically acceptable clinical trials. A major breakthrough occurred with the publication of a report in the *British Medical Journal* (2nd June 1990). The research it described was conducted by the Medical Research Council with the assistance of BCA chiropractors, and met all the conventional criteria: in a comparison between chiropractic and hospital outpatient treatment for the management of low back pain, it showed unquestionably that chiropractic was the more effective, particularly in those with long-term severe pain. A follow-up survey two years later showed that the improvements were lasting. (It should be noted, however, that the report has been criticized on the grounds that the patients receiving chiropractic treatment attended private clinics, while those receiving hospital outpatient treatment were treated under less ideal conditions.)

In 1994 the first Chiropractic Act was passed in the UK, to provide both for the regulation of chiropractic and its promotion. At the time of writing, progress is being made towards creating a single statutory register (incorporating all four of the original voluntary associations), as required by the Act, in order to regulate the profession as a whole and ensure that training standards are all equally high.

The Act has established the first General Chiropractic Council (GCC), whose membership was announced in 1997. After registration, the GCC will eventually be responsible for developing, promoting and regulating the profession of chiropractic throughout the UK, and establishing the statutory register. Once in place, it will be an offence for anyone not on this register to call him- or herself a chiropractor.

This coming together in a profession whose history has been marked by schisms and divisions represents an important landmark in the development of chiropractic in the UK – both for the professionals concerned and for the public who seek safe and effective treatment for problems which medical care has so often failed to alleviate.

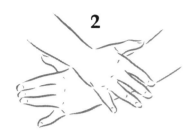

2

JOHN McTIMONEY AND
HIS SCHOOL

John McTimoney was creative, generous, unconventional,
a rebel against authority, and a gifted healer. He left a
legacy of a gentle, holistic method of manipulation whose
practitioners are steadily increasing in number and
meeting with ever-growing approval from the medical
profession.

John McTimoney's arrival on the British chiropractic
scene marked a return to the philosophy originated by D D
Palmer. Palmer's theory of Vitalism had been disputed
by scientists, and mainstream chiropractic had been
developing along scientifically-orientated lines with the
addition of tools such as X-rays. McTimoney Chiropractic,
by contrast, is in the Vitalist tradition, based on the ability
of the body's Innate Intelligence to heal itself, and follows
the belief of the 'straights' that chiropractors should assess
and treat patients using their hands alone.

Born at Edgbaston, Birmingham, on 9th March 1914, John McTimoney was the youngest of four children whose father died when he was nine months old. Although interested in healing as a child, his artistic talents led him to become an engraver. He was training as a silversmith when he met his wife Hilda; the couple moved to Oxfordshire where they worked as potters and engravers. The Depression of the 1930s ended their plans to start a jewellery-making business, so McTimoney took on other work, mainly on local farms. In 1939 a fall from a ladder forced him to give up heavy work, and during the Second World War he became a technical artist for Pressed Steel, the Ministry of Works, and the Air Ministry.

In 1942, as a result of his earlier fall, McTimoney began losing the use of his arms and experienced difficulty in walking. The only medical treatment offered was a major operation, with a 50 per cent prospect of recovery. Some years earlier, Hilda McTimoney had been cured of catarrhal deafness by a chiropractor, Mr Ashford of Birmingham, who had trained under D D Palmer. McTimoney went to Mr Ashford for treatment. Ashford's first manipulation consisted of a single adjustment to McTimoney's neck (the Hole in One treatment promulgated by B J Palmer) after which he was able to walk the five miles home. Over three years of regular treatments he was cured.

During his visits to Mr Ashford, McTimoney became fascinated by chiropractic, still a very little known therapy in Britain. He was struck by the logic of its philosophy of cause and effect, and became eager to learn it himself. At this time, however, the BCA was composed entirely of graduates from the Palmer College in Davenport who were forbidden to teach in the UK, and he could not afford to go to Iowa.

In 1944 Mr Ashford referred McTimoney to a local chiropractor, Dr Mary Walker, DC (Doctor of Chiropractic). She was a former medical nursing matron who in her fifties had trained at Palmer College under B J Palmer. In addition to chiropractic itself, she used Bach Flower Remedies, homoeopathy and radionics, as well as the neurocalometer recommended by B J to detect areas of inflammation. She had discovered, however, that her hands were more sensitive and accurate instruments for palpating and assessing misalignments.

Despite the ruling about teaching in the UK, she also hoped to start her own school of chiropractic. Her family doctor, though sympathetic, told her regretfully that he was unable to support her plan since he dared not risk being struck off. The onset of the Second World War finally put paid to her project. However, in the late 1940s she passed on her complete training, based on her meticulous notes, to her housekeeper Joan Nind (now in her seventies and still practising in Oxford). Her second pupil was John McTimoney.

McTimoney had watched her treating his family, and once when she was unavailable had actually tried out the technique for himself. He succeeded in relieving his wife of 'a very acute attack of pain and temperature with the loss of use of her left arm ... by finding which vertebra was responsible for the disorder and copying what I had witnessed so many times, adjusting the vertebrae successfully and relieving my wife to the extent that she was able to visit Dr Walker the next morning.'[1]

Needless to say, treating one's nearest and dearest without training is not generally to be recommended, but John McTimoney was particularly gifted. Recognizing his potential, Dr Walker decided to teach him herself, with two other Doctors of Chiropractic as his examiners. His training, which he described as 'comprehensive and severe', followed the curriculum of Dr Walker's planned school and took him nearly three years.

He qualified in 1950 and, in 1951, with Dr Walker's help set up what soon became a flourishing practice in Banbury. He was a dedicated therapist: stories are told of him treating people at midnight and then driving them home himself. His wife, Hilda, meanwhile continued jewellery-making, as well as raising their three children. When her arm became severely affected by neuritis, McTimoney treated her with entire success, enabling her to continue with her delicate work.

The McTimoney Technique

McTimoney's philosophy was based on D D Palmer's original discoveries and Dr Walker's teaching: that the main cause of disease and pain is the misalignment (subluxation) of bones, chiefly in the spine, which in turn interrupts the functioning of the nervous system, thus affecting general health. A subluxation may be obvious or extremely subtle, but even the latter can cause pain by compressing or stretching nerves. Adjusting the bone to its normal position thus relieves pain and returns the spine and nervous system to normal functioning; the Innate Intelligence of the body is then freed to restore health.

Constantly perfecting his technique, McTimoney developed his own method of treating the whole body, rather than simply focusing on painful areas. He realized that not just the spine but the skull, thorax, arms and legs all have joints whose bones can lose their alignment. He used his sensitive hands and fingers to analyse the skeletons of his patients in order to detect the slightest misalignment, and made gentle, subtle adjustments to restore the body's structure to normal.

Although Mary Walker had given him a full training in the techniques she had learned at the Palmer College, John McTimoney came to focus on one in particular. Mainstream chiropractors trained in the US, Canada and Bournemouth, practise what is called *diversified method*: that is, they use a variety of specific techniques for specific situations and parts of the body (*see Appendix B*). McTimoney began to refine and develop the adjustment known as the toggle-recoil, still taught at the AECC (but only to adjust the atlas, the bone supporting the skull).

The toggle-torque-recoil adjustment developed by McTimoney consists of an extremely light and fast movement. The toggle is the thrust, the torque is applied during the thrust and the recoil is the immediate removal of the practitioner's hands, allowing the patient's body to react by itself, so that the adjustment is not imposed upon it. This technique respects the body's innate knowledge of what is appropriate for it at that moment.

This adjustment is usually carried out with the hands on a specific part of the bone, usually the transverse process of a vertebra. It is a means of gently, and usually painlessly, persuading the bone to return to its correct resting position without forcing or stressing the joint or the body. Based on this principle, McTimoney developed a range of further 'sprung' adjustments which could be applied to all the joints of the body, as well as a range of direct, subtle cranial (skull) manipulations. This whole-body method of treatment (which he originally called the Palmer-McTimoney Technique) became known as the McTimoney Technique.

As time went on, McTimoney began to attract patients from all over Great Britain and abroad. Some of his difficult cases included people who were later to be influential in creating and supporting his school. Hertha Larive, for instance, later a member of the McTimoney Trust Committee of Management, came to him after visiting scores of specialists and manipulative therapists to no avail. Two childhood accidents had left her with severe scoliosis and chronic backache and headaches; later, the births of two children resulted in intermittent paralysis and chronic migraines. She was far from hopeful by the time she visited John McTimoney, on the recommendation of friends.

He palpated her spine and – though she had told him only of her back problem – gave her a history of her ailments since childhood. He explained that anyone who understood the mechanics of the spine and the nervous system could have told her as much; however, there is no doubt that he was also highly intuitive. He told her that she was one of the worst cases he had ever seen, and needed five years of regular treatments. Since she lived in Sweden, she was only able to see him for three treatments a week during three weeks a year. But following this regime for seven years saved her from life in a wheelchair.

It was Hertha Larive who introduced McTimoney to Stan Harding, later to be the McTimoney School's administrator and director. Stan Harding recalls attending a tutorial suffering from a raging toothache which had lasted several weeks and for which the dentist could find no cause. McTimoney was describing case after case of what sounded to a sceptical listener like impossible recoveries. Finally, Stan asked if chiropractic could help toothache. McTimoney examined Stan's skull, laid him on his bench with his head to the side, deftly flicked the side of his head and the pain in Stan's tooth stopped instantly.

Chiropractic for Animals

John McTimoney was by no means the first person to manipulate animals, but he claimed that his system was 'the first application of chiropractic in a complete form for animals'. This began in 1953 when one of his patients cancelled an appointment because the vet was coming to put down his seven-year-old mare: the animal had been suffering for some months from a swollen fetlock that would not respond to treatment. McTimoney, thinking this might be due to a subluxated vertebra – and that no one would put down a human being with a swollen ankle – offered to look at her. As he wrote:

Trained in human anatomy and with farming experience I adapted my knowledge of human anatomy to that of the animal, and worked out a method of adjusting the vertebrae which were subluxated ... and cured the horse in two weeks. By the end of the month the horse ... was hunting again and continued to do so for many years. At the age of 21, she was in foal.

By 1964 McTimoney was known for curing all kinds of animal disorders after normal veterinary methods had failed to help – including lameness, lack of co-ordination, and bucking and shying in horses, and lameness and 'slipped discs' in dogs. Other animals joined his patient list. Most vets, however, completely ignored his work, so for 10 years he ran into no real conflict with the veterinary profession.

Then, in 1964, when a local paper published an article about his cure of a bulldog with eczema, the Royal College of Veterinary Surgeons wrote to McTimoney pointing out that he was breaking the law by practising veterinary surgery, and could be prosecuted. McTimoney replied that he was not practising veterinary surgery but an entirely new system of animal chiropractic with which he had treated animals for 10 years with remarkable results. He invited the College to investigate his work, but the invitation was not taken up. However, his solicitors succeeded in obtaining a letter from the RCVS saying that they were prepared to regard chiropractors as physiotherapists, who are granted an exemption from the law provided they work under and with the approval of vets.

As a result of this publicity, one vet at last did show an interest – Mr E Herrod-Taylor, MRCVS, who was to become a well-known name in the field of animal manipulation. He was the first to appreciate the potential of animal chiropractic and worked with McTimoney on a number of horses. He became a proficient chiropractor himself, and he too tried to interest the veterinary profession, but with little success. Nevertheless he helped to train further McTimoney chiropractors.

McTimoney continued to treat animals, usually without a veterinary diagnosis – not for lack of effort on his part. He tried to persuade the veterinary profession that this was not a method of veterinary surgery but 'a new method which can help in cases where there is not a response to normal methods, apart from the fact that normal methods of veterinary surgery cannot help to improve the gait, movement, co-ordination, style or vices of the horse, which is what has been achieved with my methods.' But in the 1960s the general opinion was that it was impossible to manipulate a horse's spine, and that the whole thing smacked of charlatanism.

Nevertheless, McTimoney's techniques became very popular with horse owners and show jumpers, and since his day some of the horses belonging to the British Royal household have been treated by McTimoney-trained chiropractors. McTimoney's own clients included professional riders like Dorian Williams and David Broome, who later described himself as 'one of Mr McTimoney's greatest fans. He was a masterpiece ... something about the touch of his fingers was different from anybody else's. He worked wonders on Beethoven, the horse I won the World Championships on. Beethoven was going very badly one day and I took him to McTimoney. He gave him one treatment – he just knew what was going wrong. He said, "Don't jump him for four days." I jumped him on the fifth day at the Dublin Show, and he won the first two classes he entered. The man was a gem, and a gentleman with it.'

With fans like this, it is not surprising that the demand for both human and animal treatment became so great that McTimoney's health felt the strain. He suffered his first heart attack in 1969; during his convalescence his son Russell took over his practice in Banbury.

The Oxfordshire School of Chiropractic

Following this first heart attack, McTimoney was asked to take on students in order to ensure the survival of his work: this he did with his usual open-heartedness and lack of concern for finances. In 1972, with the help of his wife and his two daughters (both of whom became chiropractors), he opened the Oxfordshire School of Chiropractic, with 14 students. Animal chiropractic was included in the course; Mr Herrod-Taylor taught there for a time.

Preferring to take on mature students with some experience of life, McTimoney created a part-time course which would enable them to continue to work while studying. He assessed applicants on their personal qualities rather than their academic prowess; new applicants of whom 'Mac' approved would be taken on in mid-course.

In setting up the School, McTimoney was motivated by the desire to teach 'true chiropractic', using the hands alone. He disapproved of the medicalization of teaching in the large training schools, including the use of X-rays and stethoscopes. He wrote:

… it is my intention to teach true chiropractic, which uses only the hands, as the word chiropractic means, and relies upon no other methods of diagnosis, nor attempts to be anything but what it is. It respects the medical profession for

its own methods and does not attempt to confuse either
them or patients as to means, claims, diagnosis (or analysis),
method, etc., but relies purely upon what Palmer did,
namely, to use his hands to cure – hence the term
chiropractic. Chiropractic is a means of restoring health by
spinal manipulation and manipulation of other joints.

The three-year course consisted of monthly half-day
practical tutorials, and some 20 hours' home study a week,
50 weeks a year, covering 21 related subjects, including
anatomy, osteology and symptomatology. At his tutorials
McTimoney took students through a series of 22 exercises
aimed at producing the relaxation and flexibility required
to carry out the toggle-torque-recoil with the required
speed and thrust – perfecting the technique demands a
great deal of practice. To develop the sensitivity of their
hands in order to assess patients by palpation, students
were given such exercises as trying to palpate a hair
placed between the pages of a book through as many
pages as possible.

McTimoney taught, as D D Palmer had taught before him,
that health depends on healthy nerve messages, that
misalignments of the vertebrae or other joints interfere with
these, and that such misalignments can affect not only
joints and muscles, but every cell and organ in the body. He
also stressed what would now be called holism: that human
beings are not purely physical but mental, emotional and
spiritual beings as well, and that treating the whole body
restores health to all these aspects of the patient.

Many of McTimoney's students were wholeheartedly in
tune with this view. Stan Harding, for instance, has
commented:

Man is still a mystery. You can look at all the tissues and organs and systems of the body in a laboratory; man is much more than that. Palmer wrote that you cannot treat the body without affecting the mind and spirit. My personal belief is that a change in human consciousness can be effected by chiropractic; things actually change at a very subtle level and suddenly people see things differently. There is a known esoteric relationship between the spine and spiritual awareness. Some patients have said: 'Since I've had the treatment I've been able to manage better with my life: my perception has changed.'

The school (now College) logo, which McTimoney originally designed, depicts a drawing of Chiron, half-man, half-horse, the wisest centaur in Greek mythology. Known as the wounded healer, Chiron was not only a physician but a prophet, teacher and musician; the logo shows him carrying the torch of knowledge and the Caduceus, symbol of healing. The Latin words beneath, 'In Manu Vis Medendi', translate as 'In the hands is the power to heal'.

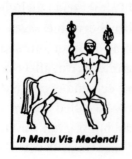

The McTimoney College logo

Two years after the school opened McTimoney suffered a second heart attack, undoubtedly brought on by overwork. This illness led to the early promotion of nine of McTimoney's advanced students (including Stan Harding and McTimoney's daughter Pauline). Those who qualified helped to treat McTimoney's own patients at Banbury, and started practices of their own. The School continued as best it could, although the animal course was temporarily dropped.

In 1980 John McTimoney died of a final heart attack at the age of 66, leaving the School to his widow. His daughters Cynthia and Pauline had been largely responsible for running it as their father's health deteriorated; after his death Pauline looked after both the administration and the teaching.

Hilda McTimoney had assumed the role of Principal, but realized she could not cope unaided. At her request the School's solicitor brought in a retired businessman, Kenneth Day, to review the situation. The report he produced stated that the Oxford School of Chiropractic had the potential to become the leader in creating a core of pure chiropractic

... if it is organized with a completely professional, and one might say, missionary approach ... John's strong character, together with his artistic nature and complete lack of interest in routine tasks, led the OSC into an utterly chaotic state ... There is a great difference between a one-man operation catering for a small number of pupils on a personal basis, of which profit was a minor consideration, and a teaching establishment providing facilities for a continuing flow of students paying substantial fees to enter a highly

*skilled profession from which they expect to receive a
satisfactory livelihood.*

The School was about to enter a new phase.

The McTimoney Chiropractic School

McTimoney's students and graduates were determined
that his work should continue. Mrs McTimoney now
turned to Stan Harding, who had already been actively
involved with training and administration. On the advice
of her solicitor, Hilda McTimoney asked him to help
reorganize the school. Stan had the advantage of being
an experienced businessman as well as a professional
chiropractor. Though already busy – running his own
business as well as working as a chiropractor – he was also
motivated by the sense of having a spiritual mission to
continue McTimoney's work. After some discussions,
he agreed to take over the running of the School, in
collaboration with Kenneth Day as business manager.

Stan Harding and a small group of supporters immediately
set about reorganizing the School along more conventional
lines. The professional association founded by McTimoney
as the John McTimoney Association of Pure Chiropractic
was re-named the Institute of Pure Chiropractic (IPC). The
School's curriculum was re-structured, and Daphne Tomlin,
a highly experienced biology teacher, was brought in to
teach anatomy and physiology. Very importantly, a group of
practising McTimoney chiropractors got together to make
detailed notes on the techniques that John McTimoney had
always kept in his brilliant but unbusinesslike head, in
order to compile a teaching manual.

By 1982, after further reorganizing and re-structuring, the school was relaunched with 18 students under the ownership of Stan Harding and McTimoney's son-in-law, Graham Wilkins. It was renamed the McTimoney Chiropractic School, in acknowledgement of the selfless work of the McTimoney family. Over the next five years Stan Harding and his dedicated team of instructors and staff continued to run the training in keeping with McTimoney's ideals, though with a much more practical emphasis (the complete history has been recorded by Stan Harding in his memoir, *McTimoney Chiropractic, the First 25 years*, to which we are indebted for much of the material in this chapter).

By 1986 McTimoney graduates represented 30 per cent of the chiropractors working in the UK, numbering 68, and the School had 70 students. In keeping with McTimoney's wish these were mature people, with the desire, motivation and determination to become McTimoney Chiropractors. Determination was needed to put in 20–30 hours' weekly study on top of their other work. The course was kept to three years, and the management team constantly worked to improve the quality of the syllabus and standards of training.

At this time the School was kept deliberately small. Although there was a greater stress on academic qualifications than before, these were not essential for entrance. The selection committee who met applicants during a day's visit to the school assessed them on their personal qualities, including their practical ability, sensitivity and potential for compassion. Ninety per cent of them were mature students who had had other careers, with a high proportion of women. Some 60 per cent were grateful patients, though some came with no experience of the technique at all, finding in the atmosphere of the School something that they had been looking for and not found elsewhere.

In 1986 Stan Harding and Graham Wilkins handed over the ownership and management of the School to the newly formed McTimoney Trust Committee of Management (CoM), peopled largely by the former committee of patrons. The animal chiropractic course was reinstated as a one-year post-graduate course, with the help of Joan Williamson from the Warwickshire College of Agriculture, who improved the syllabus. The following year Stan Harding, then in his fifties, retired. Despite health problems, he has continued to work as a skilled and dedicated chiropractor.

The McTimoney-Corley Technique

In 1986 Hugh Corley, one of McTimoney's original students, set up the Witney School of Chiropractic. Originally a farmer, he was one of McTimoney's graduates and had helped Pauline McTimoney to keep the School going during McTimoney's illness. As so often in the history of chiropractic, however, he had developed his own variations on the McTimoney technique. Eventually he set up the Oxford School of Chiropractic, teaching the McTimoney-Corley Technique. By 1998 there were around 100 practitioners on its voluntary register (the British Association for Applied Chiropractic), 125 in training, and 15 on the animal course.

Towards Recognition

Over the next few years there were a number of changes in the School's directorship, management and curriculum. The course was constantly being refined, with a view to improving educational standards and ultimately acquiring accreditation.

The 1980s saw a great expansion of interest in the complementary medical field as a whole; the public were becoming increasingly disillusioned with drug-based medicine at a time when the number of complementary practitioners in many fields was growing. At the same time, the complementary medical professions in the UK were very aware of the possible repercussions of British involvement in Europe, where different laws applied in different countries, and some therapies were illegal in some places. The McTimoney School management realized, as the numbers of students, practitioners and patients increased, the necessity of joining the general move among the complementary medical professions to set their houses in order and agree on acceptable standards of training, ethics and practice.

Bodies like the Council for Complementary and Alternative Medicine were being set up with the aim of helping reputable therapies to achieve recognition. The therapies represented by the CCAM were well established: acupuncture, BCA chiropractic, homoeopathy, medical herbalism, naturopathy and osteopathy. At this time, the BCA objected to the inclusion of the IPC – and indeed to its use of the word 'chiropractic', since McTimoney Chiropractic differed substantially from that practised by the BCA. Moreover, it was taught part-time over three years, by comparison with the AECC's full-time, four-year, academically-orientated course.

After taking legal advice, the IPC stuck to the use of the word 'chiropractic'. It also launched in 1991 a new four-year course. The previous year the British government had stated that if the chiropractic profession was to be recognized, chiropractors must present a united front. Dialogues between the IPC and BCA over the years had already been leading to greater understanding, and the BCA recognized that a four-year course along Open University lines was acceptable.

Thus the 1990s saw serious expansion and forward movement for the School and the IPC. In 1992 the Royal College of Veterinary Surgeons accepted the McTimoney Animal Manipulation Course, which in turn agreed to accept non-McTimoney trained veterinary students, and McTimoney chiropractors began to attend equine events.

The technique was proving as popular as ever, and gaining in recognition as a safe and valid therapy for problems that medicine was still failing to relieve – an article in *The Daily Mail* produced no fewer than 6,000 enquiries, and would-be students were writing in from all over the world. In December 1994 the Clinical Standards Advisory Group, an independent multi-disciplinary group commissioned by the UK Department of Health, recommended that doctors should send appropriate patients with low back pain to chiropractors and members of other recognized manipulative professions. Doctors were showing an increased interest in the therapy: McTimoney chiropractors began to be invited to work within one or two medical practices. An informal patient survey carried out in 1997 showed that 89 per cent of respondents were extremely or very satisfied with their treatment.

The real watershed, however, was the passage of Chiropractic Act in 1994. This put an obligation on all branches of chiropractic to join forces in order to produce a statutory national register of practitioners (replacing the four voluntary registers), and to agree on acceptable, and as far as possible uniform, standards of training and practice.

Also in 1994, two changes of name marked what was to be a new era in the history of McTimoney Chiropractic: the IPC was renamed the McTimoney Chiropractic Association (MCA) and the School became the McTimoney Chiropractic College (MCC). Full weekend courses were introduced to the syllabus, and it was decided for the first time to bring in a Principal whose background was not in chiropractic but in education: Ian Pearson, who joined the College in 1995 and produced a plan for achieving degree status. Negotiations with the University of Wales, meanwhile, reached agreement for the validation of the human training course, now designated Diploma of Higher Education in McTimoney Chiropractic; this was followed in 1997 by validation of the animal course by the University of Wales and the Warwick College of Agriculture as a post-graduate diploma course – the only externally validated post-graduate course in animal manipulation.

In addition to the distance-learning course at the Abingdon College, a full-time course was launched in the autumn of 1998 at the University of Westminster. This three-year course leads to a BSc Honours degree in Health Sciences, with a year's post-graduate chiropractic diploma, with McTimoney Chiropractic as the chiropractic pathway. Most of the teaching takes place in London, but students also visit the McTimoney Chiropractic College in Abingdon regularly, particularly for practical sessions and clinical practice.

At the end of 1998, the Principal Ian Pearson resigned, having achieved his aims for the College in getting the McTimoney courses validated. Practising chiropractor Dr Christina Cunliffe took over as Principal. Dr Cunliffe is also a Doctor of Philosophy in the Life Sciences, a Chartered Biologist and a Member of the Institute of Biology, and has gained financial, business management and marketing experience at senior levels in the information industry. Dr Cunliffe's experience both in business and chiropractic makes her particularly suited to lead the College into its next phase.

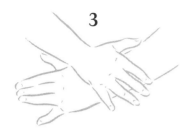

3

McTIMONEY COLLEGE
TRAINING

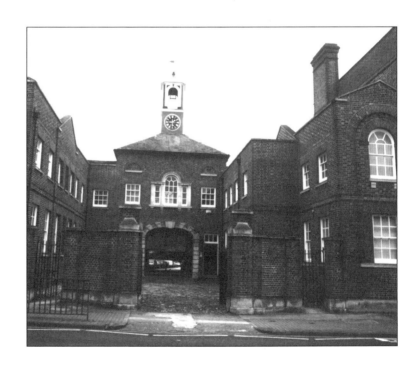

The Clock House

The McTimoney Chiropractic College

The College is now located at the Clock House in Abingdon, Oxfordshire. The premises include three clinic rooms for treating patients and for students' clinical practice. Its equipment is modern, including such facilities as a video link enabling students to observe practitioners at work without intruding on their patients, and access to a library in Oxford with CD ROM and Internet links.

The four-year Diploma of Higher Education, validated by the University of Wales and launched in January 1997, is a far cry from John McTimoney's original, highly personal approach. It has changed as a result of the need to achieve the standards required for registration. As a distance learning course (with a high proportion of contact time) it attracts mature, experienced people with a sense of vocation, since it is flexible enough to allow them to continue their careers while training.

An outline of the curriculum is given on pages 44–5: as you can see, it covers a wide range of subjects, taught on a modular basis, from the theoretical to the practical. The 50 or so part-time tutors who deliver the course, form a multi-disciplinary team, many being specialists in subjects outside chiropractic. Students are therefore exposed to a broad range of views on health and health-related subjects. Throughout the course there is an average staff-student ratio of one to four for practical training, and it is not unusual to have a ratio of one to two in clinics. The administration and teaching involves over 100 members of staff in all, mainly part-time.

McTimoney Students

The total number of students is about 180, with an annual entry of around 50. The minimum age of entry is 18, but the majority are mature students, typically in their early thirties, and with a higher proportion of women than men. They are required to have the standard higher education entrance qualifications, but those without degrees or the requisite A-levels do have other options such as an APEL (Approved Prior Experiential Learning) system of assessment, now used by most universities, and an Access Course. Applicants are also assessed on their personal qualities for – to quote the College prospectus – 'their sense of vocation, motivation, and qualities of determination and aspiration'.

Determination and aspiration are essential: although the course is not officially full-time, the actual amount of time entailed amounts to more than some 'full-time' courses. The McTimoney training demands a good 20 hours a week of home study and practice. On-site tutorials, formerly one day a month, now take up a full weekend each month, and since 1997 a summer school has also formed part of the course in the first two years. Students begin observing in clinics from the first year, and by the third and fourth years clinical work may demand one day's attendance a week.

What has not changed since John McTimoney's time is an atmosphere of enthusiasm and dedication among the students, buoyed up by the knowledge that they are embarking on a very worthwhile career, together with a sense of camaraderie and mutual support.

Human Chiropractic Course

Year 1

Functional Anatomy I - Bones and Joints

Functional Anatomy II - Myology, Biomechanics and Movement

Human Physiology I*

Biochemistry, Histology

Philosophy and Ethics

Complementary Therapies*

Functional Anatomy III - (Neuroanatomy)

Practical Studies (College)

Practical Studies (Summer School)*

Research Methods and Special Topic*

Personal and Professional Development

Clinic Placement

Seminar Programme

Tutorials*

Year 2

Imaging Techniques

Orthopaedics

Physiology II

Biomechanics II and III

Patient Communication I

Health and Hygiene

Behavioural Sciences*

Complementary Therapies* + Clinic Introduction*

Pathology and Laboratory Diagnostics*

Practical Studies (College)

Practical Studies (Summer School)*

Genetics and Embryology

Pharmacology

Personal and Professional Development

Clinic Placement - Observation and Clinic Journal Research

Seminar Programme

Tutorials*

The College curriculum

Year 3

Differential Diagnosis and
  Contraindications

Clinical Neurology (including
  Neurological Assessment)

Rheumatic Diseases

Radiology and Imaging
  Interpretation

Patient Communication II

Nutrition

Practical Studies

Pathology

Personal and Professional
  Development

Clinic Practice

Seminar Programme

Year 4

Practice Management and
  Private Practice Start Up

Orthopaedic Testing

Gynaecology

Obstetrics

Paediatrics

Geriatrics

Dermatology

Research Methodology and
  Clinic Project

Models of Public Health/NHS
  GP Fund Holding

Practical Studies

Personal and Professional
  Development

Clinic Practice

Seminar Programme

* Included in summer school programme

What kind of people choose to undertake four years of hard work – six in the case of those who train as animal manipulators? Most of these mature students are going through a major change of direction in life: they may, for example, be tired of offices and office politics, and want a more human approach to working with people. Some may have been made redundant, though most will continue in their paid work while studying. Some are qualified therapists in other fields, including medicine, nursing and occupational health – people whose desire to relieve the pain of others has been frustrated in the orthodox field – as well as complementary therapists who want to broaden their range of treatments. The majority will have experienced the benefits of McTimoney treatment for their own problems or those of people near to them. People aiming to do the animal course will almost certainly have seen the benefits to both horses and riders.

There is, however, a difference between today's student intake and that of even 10 years ago: while many students have been drawn to the technique through personal experience, a number of current students have also looked very thoroughly into all the available manipulative courses before opting for the McTimoney College. For some the main appeal is the flexibility that enables them to study while still earning. In addition, the College's academic record is increasingly well regarded, and its facilities compare well with other part-time colleges.

Skilful Hands

There is an ongoing debate within the complementary therapy professions as to whether the emphasis on intellectual knowledge demanded by the new rules for registration may detract from the qualities that patients value in their therapists: humanity, compassion – and, of course, practical, effective treatment. In fact aptitude is absolutely essential: academic knowledge is not acquired at the expense of technique.

The physical practice of the McTimoney techniques begins in the first year, and from then on students are expected to practise specific exercises daily in order to build up the right muscles and flexibility and to develop the manual sensitivity required for expert palpation. The toggle-torque-recoil technique on which most adjustments are based (*see Chapter 2* and *Appendix B*) requires as much accuracy and expertise as it ever did, and the McTimoney style of assessment requires the ability to detect bones even very subtly out of place throughout the whole body.

Today's curriculum includes radiology – the ability to understand X-rays and MRI scans and the reports accompanying them from the chiropractic point of view. In John McTimoney's time the view was that 'If you can't palpate it, you can't adjust it,' while McTimoney himself was wary of the possible harm caused by X-rays. Today, while it is acknowledged that useful information can be found in the many techniques of imaging now available, the main purpose of sending a chiropractic patient for X-ray is to rule out underlying pathology such as metasteses and arthritic conditions. Chiropractors may find them particularly useful with patients who have suffered severe accidents or surgery, or in whom arthritis of the spine may be a factor.

Students are also taught to be aware that not all back and joint pains stem from the musculo-skeletal system; they may be related, for instance, to heart problems, diabetes, kidney or gall-bladder malfunction, and some forms of cancer. As many patients are self-referred and may not have had a medical check-up, practitioners have to be alert to the possibility that a patient may turn up with an undiagnosed medical condition. They are trained to detect, from the patient's general health and other symptoms, whether a serious condition is present, and to refer patients back to their doctors or to other specialists if there is the slightest indication of such a problem.

Unique Features

One of the unique features of McTimoney Chiropractic is the depth at which practitioners are taught sensitivity of touch and palpation skills, which probably exceeds that of any of the other manipulative therapies.

These skills are such that McTimoney chiropractors have been known to correct erroneous medical diagnoses by touch alone, as in the case of one patient whose medically diagnosed 'multiple sclerosis' symptoms turned out to be caused by a subluxated vertebra in the neck causing pressure on the spinal cord, which the chiropractor was able to treat. 'The most common medical "misdiagnosis", says one, is "you'll just have to live with it!" when in fact the patient's pain can be cured by adjustment.'

In the UK there are three McTimoney clinics where students gain clinical experience, first by observation and then, in the third and fourth year, under supervision, with a unique tutor-student ratio of as little as one to two. One clinic is within the College building, and the others are at York and Northampton.

Holism: Mind, Body and Spirit

The appeal of the McTimoney training has always been its holistic approach. Caring for the whole person – mind, body and spirit – is one of the factors that draws patients to most complementary therapies as opposed to orthodox medical care.

The concept of holism, and of the need to acknowledge the spirit as much as the body, goes back to the philosophy of Palmer and was an essential ingredient of John McTimoney's teaching. Today, in the much more practical environment of the College and its teaching, this has not been so much lost as up-dated: John McTimoney's teachings were in tune with his times, the 1960s and 1970s. The terminology of the 1990s is perforce more scientifically based, but this does not mean that the spirit has been lost.

The curriculum includes modules on chiropractic Philosophy and Ethics, including Palmer's belief in Innate and Universal Intelligence. It is becoming much more widely accepted in the field of health-care, both orthodox and complementary, that patients' attitudes and emotional stresses have an important effect on their bodily health. In the McTimoney curriculum these factors are addressed by subjects such as Sociology and Psychology, which form an important part of the course. The Behavioural Sciences module covers basic counselling, and referring patients for professional counselling when necessary. Practitioners who are dealing directly with people's bodies need to understand the role played by the mind and the emotions, as well as by social stresses and environmental factors, and to recognize when other forms of therapy may be needed.

In any form of health-care the quality of the practitioner-patient relationship is crucial: the medical profession itself acknowledges that the doctor's manner towards his or her patients and belief in the treatment offered can affect the course of recovery. With hands-on, physical treatments, patients need to have total trust in their therapists. One of the advantages of taking in mature students is that most will have already experienced the importance of interpersonal skills during their working life, and have an interest in developing these. The McTimoney curriculum includes modules on Patient Communication, as well as Personal and Professional Development. Clinical practice, and observing experienced chiropractors at work, provides further training in these areas as well as the ethical aspects of the work – including tact, being aware of other people's boundaries and respecting patients' confidentiality.

The Practitioner's Outlook

There is another, less tangible aspect of holistic treatment which does not appear in the curriculum. Behind every adjustment there is something not easily definable or testable: the chiropractor's unspoken attitude and beliefs, his or her desire to heal, and his or her rapport with the patient.

There are some McTimoney practitioners whose approach can be called spiritual, or at least strongly intuitive. This is also true of therapists in other forms of complementary medicine, who are often involved in forms of self-development such as meditation. One-to-one treatment in a quiet setting can create an atmosphere which allows the intuition to emerge, so that practitioners may find themselves successfully treating someone by inspiration rather than literally and slavishly by the book.

These are skills that are not and cannot be taught in an academically-oriented curriculum. They develop over time through experience and personal development: they are creative skills, and as with other forms of creativity are best backed with a good grounding in technique and practice.

Graduation and Post-graduate Studies

The training described here aims to produce well-rounded, knowledgeable and skilful practitioners. Practical elements include modules on running a practice, such as how to set up in partnership, acquiring equipment, the legal side, insurance, how to keep books for tax returns, and of course keeping good patient records.

Students are assessed throughout by methods appropriate to the subjects, including written examinations, projects, oral presentations and of course practical assessment. While the first year is set above A-level standards, the course progresses quickly to degree level work, and students' progress is constantly monitored. At the end of four years and a satisfactory assessment of students' knowledge and abilities, they are awarded a Practitioner's Certificate, and can become associate members of the

McTimoney Chiropractic Association, the professional body which governs the Code of Ethics and has – up until the enforcement of the Chiropractic Act in 1999 – maintained the register of practitioners.

By the time they graduate, these newly qualified chiropractors will have become experienced in dealing with patients. During the last three months, those who have passed their final examination are qualified and insured to work with members of the public (either from their own homes or within a local practice) and can charge a small fee. They are required to fill out record cards for new patients which are vetted by mentors (practising chiropractors who are usually in the same area). These mentors also vet the students' letters to the doctors of new patients, and can advise on any problems that may arise during the course of a treatment. In this way, by the time they leave the College, novice chiropractors will have become acclimatized to taking responsibility for patient management, and will have a dozen or more patients on their books.

Under the Chiropractic Act 1994 newly qualified chiropractors are required to complete a Provisional Registration Year (PRY) during which they continue their development and education. The McTimoney Chiropractic Association (MCA) already had this system in place, since it has for many years required new graduates to complete an Associate programme which includes advanced chiropractic techniques and other aspects of the professional management of patients and practices. Other post-graduate courses are to be developed in the future.

Some graduates choose to add other skills and techniques to their repertoire which are not offered by the College curriculum. These include such subjects as counselling, nutrition, soft tissue work, polarity therapy and Applied Kinesiology (which aids both assessment and treatment by the use of muscle-testing techniques).

The Animal Course

The post-graduate course which radically distinguishes the McTimoney training from others is, of course, the training in Animal Manipulation. The two-year Diploma in Animal Manipulation was launched in January 1998. In designing the course, the McTimoney College has worked closely with the Royal College of Veterinary Surgeons. The tutors now number animal experts from other disciplines, including vets and lecturers from Warwick College.

The course itself is open not only to qualified McTimoney chiropractors but to BSc graduates (Hons) in appropriate subjects (Animal Science, Equine Science, etc.), and to manipulators in other fields such as osteopathy, physiotherapy and other forms of chiropractic; at the request of the RCVS it is also open to vets. All applicants must have previous experience with animals, evidenced by such qualifications as a British Horse Society Stage I and II (Horse and Management) award or Pony Club B Test; those without formal animal training can submit a portfolio of certified experience for consideration.

Still run as a distance-learning course, and comprising substantial work, the first year covers theory (covering such subjects as animal anatomy, physiology and pathology as well as philosophy and ethics) and is held mainly at Warwick College whose facilities at Moreton Morrell include access to farm and domestic animals. The second year is devoted to practical experience with animals.

McTimoney Chiropractic and the Medical Profession

The McTimoney ethos has always encouraged chiropractors to develop and maintain good relations with the medical profession. The Chiropractic Act 1994 has been designed to protect the public by establishing a statutory register of chiropractors. We may hope that it will also benefit both chiropractors and doctors by increasing medical awareness of the possibilities of chiropractic.

Back pain is one of the major health problems in the West today, and one of the least well served by orthodox medicine. Doctors themselves are only too aware of this, but do not always have the knowledge – or the trust – to refer patients to non-medical manipulative therapists.

The attitude of the medical profession towards complementary therapies has been undergoing a quiet revolution over the last two decades. A British Medical Association report in 1993 accepted that there is a widespread use of non-conventional therapies, though stressing the need to protect the public against unskilled or unscrupulous practitioners, and for non-conventional therapies to be properly regulated. According to this report, nearly three-quarters of British doctors had referred patients to a non-conventional therapist at some time, and 80 per cent of a sample of medical students expressed a wish to train in one or more non-conventional therapies. As of late 1998, 40 per cent of doctors offer some form of complementary therapy through their surgeries, while 70 per cent refer patients to complementary practitioners.

A number of doctors have started referring people after having had their attention drawn to chiropractic through reports from satisfied patients. Most are likely to send them along the conventional medical route first, and obtain the opinions of orthopaedic surgeons or physiotherapists, together with any necessary investigations such as X-rays, before referring them for manipulation.

With medicine largely unable to cope with back pain, while the manipulative therapies including McTimoney Chiropractic are demonstrating good results, there is in theory one obvious solution: to make chiropractic available in Britain on the National Health Service. If some means could be found for the NHS to fund appropriate referrals to chiropractors (and, indeed, to osteopaths and other complementary therapists), the cost should be well outweighed by the fact that patients with spinal problems would be treated more quickly and might actually get better, instead of returning time after time to see doctors who are unable to help them; it would also reduce the cost to the nation as the result of loss of working days through sickness. And patients themselves would receive speedy, expert treatment and relief from pain, a benefit which cannot be measured financially.

There is clearly a major gap in health care, and whatever the financial and logistical difficulties, urgent

consideration should be given to providing skilled and
expert treatment to all back sufferers at as early a stage as
possible, before their problems become chronic.

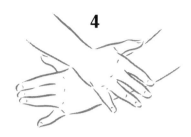

4

THE McTIMONEY
TREATMENT

Finding a McTimoney Chiropractor

People visit chiropractors for many reasons. They may
have had a good recommendation from a friend or from
their doctor or complementary medicine practitioner
who has a good reciprocal understanding with a local
chiropractor. If you have none of these, you can apply
to the McTimoney Chiropractic Association (MCA)
for the Practitioners Register or to ask for the address
of your nearest practitioner, or find a list in your local
Yellow Pages.

The MCA regulates its qualified practitioners and
standards of professionalism, which guarantees quality of
care. It is not advisable to visit an unqualified manipulator
about whom you know nothing, as English law does not at
present prevent anyone from calling themselves a

chiropractor (this will change in 1999, when the General Chiropractic Council registration comes into force).

Times and Fees

Treatment times are generally one hour for a first visit, and half to three-quarters of an hour for follow-up treatments. Fees will vary accordingly, and as with many other professions, tend to be higher in London. Always ask before you make an appointment. Some practitioners are able to use discretion in cases of hardship or when treating children.

The first visit is necessarily longer because the practitioner will need to take a complete history of your problem. At this visit, because many people are unfamiliar with chiropractic, an explanation is given of chiropractic and what you are likely to experience in a treatment. This is also the opportunity for you to ask all the questions you want before committing yourself to receiving treatment.

The complete history of your problem may be far wider and more detailed than you expect. It includes your 'presenting symptoms' (those you feel now), past accidents and operations, your general medical history and your family medical history. Your practitioner may also like to look at any previous X-rays, so if you have them, take them along with you.

The Specific Problem

Your practitioner will want to know how long you have been suffering from this problem, what you think was the cause, how long ago it happened and what you were doing when it occurred, where you feel pain now and what it stops or hinders you from doing. He or she will also want to know what eases the pain and what makes it worse, whether you have had it or something like it before, whether it is getting worse or receding (and how quickly), what time of day the pain is at its worst, and if it wakes you at night or stops you sleeping. The area of pain will be noted on your patient record card.

The dimensions, consistency and type of pain are also important: Is it deep or closer to the surface of your skin? Does it move about or stay in the same place? Is it a shooting, throbbing, stabbing, burning pain or a dull ache? The level of pain on a scale of 10 is useful to know (with 0 being no pain, 10 the worst pain you can imagine). The clearer and more specific you can be about your problem, the easier it is to define and to refer back to at a later date. It is very easy to forget just how bad a pain was, once it has gone. If you have more than one area of pain, keep the descriptions separate, because separate problems may clear up at different rates.

Contributing Factors

Often, forgotten incidents are predisposing factors to a pain: past similar accidents or unresolved problems, operation scars nearby – which are accidents in the body's terms – all add up to a possibly minor incident setting off the pain. For instance, the effects of childhood falls may have appeared to have cleared up long ago, but there may be a residual misalignment which, because body tolerances are wide in childhood, caused no pain at the time. In later life, however, a person's posture is usually worse and joints have become stiffer; consequently you feel stiffness and/or pain. You may wonder where it came from without realizing where it originated.

Your practitioner will want to know what sports and hobbies you engage in, as well as the warm-up/cool-down and flexibility exercises you practise. If you take part in competitive sport, the practitioner will also want to know if you are over-trained and stale or lack adequate endurance training for your sports schedule.

What you do at work may be relevant, especially if you do a lot of lifting, sitting, travelling or repetitive movements.

It is also worth noting that pain levels tend to increase as stress levels rise. We all have optimum stress levels, and too little stress can be as bad for the body as too much. You may be bored and have too much time to worry about your pain, or you may be pushing yourself towards burnout, so that the pain you feel is a warning sign.

The aim of history-taking is, of course, to find out about your specific problem, but it is also to eliminate pathology such as fractures, tumours and infection. Treatment is contra-indicated in these cases, and if any of these underlying problems are suspected you will be referred back to your doctor for further diagnostic tests, X-ray or scan. No treatment will be given until these signs and symptoms are resolved to your doctor's satisfaction. You may also be referred back to your doctor for other investigative tests to eliminate conditions that should be resolved before chiropractic treatment is started. If McTimoney chiropractic is unsuitable for your condition, you may also be referred to a more appropriate practitioner.

Frequently childhood illnesses such as measles, chicken pox, rubella and mumps leave a residual weakness. There may also be inherited family weaknesses – typically, several close relatives may all have suffered from chest or heart complaints, or cancer. It is important to know about these to alert your practitioner to look out for early signs or possible contra-indications to treatment, and to warn you and your doctor.

You will be asked about the functioning of the main internal organs of your body, because this provides an indication of the general functioning of your nervous system. It often happens that patients report that although they came for one complaint which has then cleared, other less severe complaints such as headaches or menstrual problems have cleared as well. This is due to the general improvement in the state of the nervous system and reduction in pain and other stress levels effected by chiropractic.

All of the different parts of your medical history will be considered by your practitioner, but you will not be given a 'diagnosis' in the medical sense. Your condition will be seen as a whole-body state of dis-ease and dysfunction, not a named disease at a specific location. The aim of the treatment is not to fight off something that has attacked you from without, but to restore you to a state of normal good function and to promote your health and self-care so that your innate healing ability (the same ability that heals cuts and grazes) will heal you, *by itself*.

After the history-taking, and if the practitioner feels McTimoney chiropractic can help you, he or she will then explain what the treatment consists of, and how the nervous system supplies all areas of the body. You will be told that you will receive a whole-body skeletal check at every treatment, but that adjustments will only be made as needed.

Assessment is carried out both while seated and lying down, and will include the whole body, not just the area of pain. One reason for this is the possibility of compensation – the body's short-term coping mechanism for any misalignment or joint stiffness. If, for example, the pelvis is tilted, the body does its best to straighten itself out, so that you can always relate to the level horizon (which is sensed by nervous responses from your eyes, ears and postural muscles – especially in the neck). The longer the original problem has been ongoing, the more compensation there has to be to cope (that is, the more other parts of your body have to tilt and the more misalignment or stiffness there is).

Since the treatment works *with* your body and does not impose adjustments upon it, where a misalignment does not reduce immediately there will be no attempt to force it into alignment. Sometimes the body has its own priorities, and needs time to undo what can sometimes be many years' structural compensation for a misalignment problem.

It is very common for a scoliosis (S-shaped spine) to straighten when the cause of the problem is removed. If the pain area alone were treated, the compensatory scoliosis (and with it the pain) would simply recur. When the cause is removed the compensatory scoliosis then does not return, and nor does the pain.

What Does the Treatment Feel Like?

As explained earlier, the McTimoney treatment uses a particularly fast and light type of adjustment known as a toggle-torque-recoil. The speed of adjustment overcomes any muscle tension and fear the patient may have. The torque means that the line of drive is focused on one spot, and the recoil ensures that the chiropractor's hands are already off the patient's body before they have had time to stop any natural rebound of the bone in question back into a more normal position. Pain, if it does occur, is only momentary. The biggest response to an adjustment is often just surprise that it's already over so quickly.

All of the many McTimoney adjustments are 'sprung' in this way, which means that no adjustments are forced or imposed upon the patient's body, and 'cavitation' noises such as a click or crunch are extremely unlikely. Patients find this type of treatment particularly comfortable to receive and very quickly relax, which makes adjustment even easier for the practitioner. The lightness of treatment surprises many patients (particularly those expecting a heavier type of adjustment) and this also means that it is particularly suitable for the very sensitive, the elderly and even children and babies.

How Often and How Many Treatments Will I Need?

Some forms of chiropractic require several treatments a week to begin with. McTimoney treatments, in contrast to most other manipulative modalities, are spaced a minimum of one week apart. This allows for any reactions occurring within the first 48 hours to subside. The next three or four days often show an improvement and then, as the week ends, the patient may experience a mild relapse due to the way the body is being used in daily life in the intervening days. It is at this point that the next treatment is needed. When the patient has been pain-free for a week, the time between treatments is increased to 14 days and then one month, the intervals increasing each time, until this pain-free state becomes the norm. By this point the patient will be more aware of his or her body's needs and may well wish only to come back every three to six months for a check (particularly if the problem is occupationally related), rather as one does with the dentist.

Three Stages of Healing

There are three basic stages to healing through chiropractic. In stage one the cause of the problem is found and the pain reduced. This stage may involve 'retracing' – where, as each layer of mechanical stress and compensation is removed, patterns of old aches and pains not felt for many years may show up again, ready to be sorted out.

Stage two involves observation of habitual and unconscious body use of both the self and other people, exercise and learning how to balance one-sided body use. It is vital to recognize, undo and counteract those postural patterns of body use inherent in specific activities. These may range from the unconscious habit of putting more weight on one leg while waiting for something (e.g. in a checkout queue, at a bus stop, at a party, while shaving, when doing the washing up, raking the lawn, vacuuming, etc.) to occupational problems such as always twisting the same way to answer the telephone or having your paperwork always on the same side of your keyboard, and hobbies or pursuits which use the body asymmetrically such as playing golf or cricket, or practising the violin.

Stage three is the three- to six-monthly check-up when you are mostly in control of your own posture and body use, but want to catch any slight misalignments while they are still easily reversible.

How many visits you will need depends upon three main factors: how long you have had the problem (rule of thumb is one month's treatment for every year you have had the problem); your age – younger people are more flexible and heal faster; and finally, your sense of responsibility and willingness to help yourself by applying some basic rules and doing the exercises you are given.

If there has been absolutely no change in your condition after six to ten treatments, your practitioner may decide that McTimoney may not be the best method of treatment for you to pursue. However, by then he or she will probably know where best to refer you, for instance back to your doctor, to a nutritionist, to an Alexander Technique teacher, or to an acupuncturist.

Reactions

After your first (and maybe your second) treatment you will be reminded about possible reactions. Most reactions are slight; they are mentioned here just to reassure you and forestall worry.

Despite the gentleness of the technique, during a course of treatment most patients will feel changes in their structure as the skeleton is realigned to remove interference to nerve fibres. Following a session it is a good idea to take the rest of the day gently, and avoid strenuous, demanding or stressful activity.

Reactions can vary from slight stiffness, soreness or a feeling of having done a 'workout' to tiredness, poor concentration or irritability. Only about 40 per cent of people have adverse reactions, and probably the most common response is tiredness. Some people report a sense of euphoria and well-being.

Whether you have a reaction or not bears no relation to the efficacy of the treatment, or to age, gender or body size – frail old ladies have been known to feel bright and perky after a treatment, and big husky he-men to feel as if they have been flattened by a steamroller!

You may be tempted to have a long hot soak in the bath after a treatment to try to ease stiffness. This is counterproductive. Continued heat causes ligament laxity, aggravates any inflammation or swelling you may have had beforehand, and allows the body to revert to its old protective or compensatory pre-treatment position. There is of course no reason why you should not have a quick shower or bath, however!

What Do Practitioners Do in a Treatment?

The McTimoney treatment is a top-to-toe regime in which the practitioner uses his or her hands only, making use of his or her finely tuned sense of touch (palpation). Superficially it may seem as though the treatment is methodically the same each time. This is far from the truth. The 'treatment flow' (order in which treatment takes place) is there to make sure everything is checked in order and nothing gets forgotten, but each treatment is individual. The practitioner treats only the misalignments found that day, and only adjusts where adjustment is needed. This means there are no extraneous adjustments. The aim is to check the alignment of the main joints and to mobilize the smaller joints to ensure that (a) there is no hindrance to correct nerve flow to each and every part of the body, and (b) that the body is free to move in any direction from a centre of correct alignment and balance.

After taking the detailed history already described, you may be offered a gown to wear and will be asked to undress down to your underwear, and to remove any jewellery, glasses or wristwatch. A typical treatment flow starts with the chiropractor standing behind the seated patient and palpating (feeling) the position of the atlas (C1) under the ears at the very top of the neck. The practitioner then proceeds down the back of the neck (C2–7). Next the back is palpated from top to bottom (T1–L5), the pelvic (hip) bones are checked for height difference between each side, and finally muscle bulk and general sitting posture are observed.

Next you will be asked to lie on your side; your atlas and neck vertebrae will be adjusted as appropriate. Your position will be changed to supine (lying on your back) and your lying posture will be observed, the slack taken out of your buttock muscles and your leg lengths checked. In the light of what is found, the practitioner will move to the pelvis and adjust it to correct tilt, rotation and torque. He or she will then move to your knees, shins and feet,

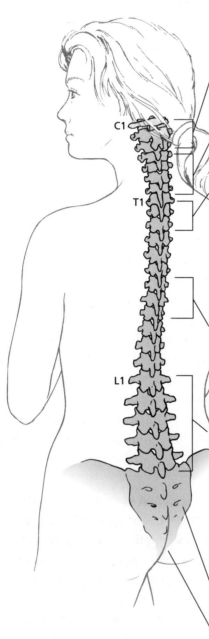

C1 - Blood supply to the head, pituitary gland, scalp, bones of the face, brain, inner end middle ear, sympathetic nervous system, eyes

C2 - Eyes, optic nerves, auditory nerves, sinuses, mastoid bones, tongue, forehead, heart

C3 - Cheeks, outer ear, face, bones, teeth, trifacial nerve, lungs

C4 - Nose, lips, mouth, Eustachian tube, mucus membranes, lungs

C5 - Vocal cords, neck glands, pharynx

C6 - Neck muscles, shoulders, tonsils

C7 - Thyroid gland, bursa in the shoulders, elbow

TI - Arms from the elbows down, including hands, arms, wrist and fingers; oesophagus and trachea; heart

T2 - Heart, including its valves and covering; coronary arteries, lungs, bronchial tubes

T3 - Lungs, bronchial tubes, pleura, chest, breast, heart

T4 - Gall bladder and common duct

T5 - Liver, solar plexus

T6 - Stomach

T7 - Pancreas, duodenum, stomach, liver, spleen, gall bladder, peritoneum

T8 - Spleen, stomach, liver, pancreas, gall bladder, adrenal cortex, small intestine, pyloric valve, diaphragm

T9 - Adrenal cortex, pancreas, spleen gall bladder, ovaries, uterus, small intestine

T10 - Kidneys, abdominal muscles

T11 - Kidneys, ureter, abdominal muscles

T12 - Small intestine, Fallopian tubes, lymph circulation

LI - Large intestine, inguinal rings, uterus

L2 - Appendix, abdomen, upper leg, urinary bladder

L3 - Sex organs, uterus, bladder, knees prostate, large intestine

L4 - Prostate gland, muscles of the lower back, sciatic nerve

L5 - Lower legs, ankles, feet, prostate

Sacrum - Hip bones, buttocks, rectum, sex organs, genitalia, urinary bladder, ureter, prostate

Coccyx - Rectum, anus

The Essentials of McTimoney Chiropractic

checking both alignment and mobilization. Arms, elbows, wrists and hands are then checked, followed by the facial bones. Checking the alignment of the collar bones and ribs completes this stage.

You will then be asked to lie prone (on your front) and the spine will be rechecked from the base of the neck to the coccyx (tail bone). The reason for this second check is that, when in this position, the spine does not have to compensate for pelvic misalignments, since it is horizontal and unaffected by gravity in the normal way. Frequently, where the spine shows a scoliosis when vertical (e.g. when sitting) and before pelvic adjustment, it will now be straight. This clearly shows that the scoliosis was just a compensation for pelvic misalignments and the vertebrae are not at fault themselves, and thus do not need to be adjusted. While you are still lying prone, the backs of the ribs, the back of the pelvis, the sacrum and coccyx are all checked and adjusted as necessary, and a three-stage massage is performed over the entire back to bring blood to the surface to assist the healing process.

Finally you will be asked to sit up again. The occiput (back of the head) and the shoulder joints are checked and the entire spine rechecked and compared with the original findings at the start of the treatment.

All adjustments throughout the entire treatment are recorded to ensure continuity. The chiropractor may give you a summary of the main findings and will probably discuss your posture and may give you appropriate exercises. These aspects of your treatment are described in Chapter 6.

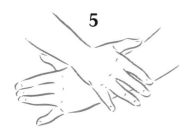

5

WHAT CAN McTIMONEY CHIROPRACTIC HELP?

Chiropractors tend to be known as people who treat backs – perhaps because so many people suffer from back pain. Yet you will know after reading the preceding chapters that chiropractic treats the whole body and all kinds of ailments. It has done so since Palmer's first treatment of Harvey Lillard. As patients with accidents and injuries, headaches and migraine, sciatica and digestive troubles responded to his treatment, Palmer realized he had discovered something far-reaching. Today chiropractic is the most popular alternative to drugs and surgery in the world. This chapter discusses some of the most common problems helped by chiropractic, with some case histories (with names omitted) to show you the scope of this wonderful treatment.

The main cause of misalignment of any part of your body lies in the way that that part, and the body as a whole, has been used (hence the strong emphasis on guided self-help in Chapter 6). According to one pain authority, J Mannheim MD, 'Bad posture and body mechanics are the most overlooked causes of musculo-skeletal pain.'[1]

The Spine and Nervous System

The spine is the lifeline of the body, because running through it is the spinal cord, a cable-like structure containing billions of nerve fibres that receive and send or carry messages to and from every part of the body. The whole skeletal system is designed for flexibility and strength. As long as the vertebrae and joints remain in good alignment, these functions are fulfilled.

The spinal column is composed of 24 vertebrae, with the sacrum and coccyx below and the cranium above, protecting the spinal cord and brain respectively (see illustration on 4, page 68). The shoulder and pelvic girdles, ribs, arms and hands, legs and feet protect the peripheral nervous system; they hang from the spine, the central or axial part of the skeleton.

Each of the 24 vertebrae can move in six different directions – forward or backward, tilted left or right, and rotating to the left or right.

The many joints in the skeleton thus allow great flexibility, and no harm comes from normal bending, stretching and twisting. When you perform these, each vertebra moves slightly in relation to its neighbours. However, forced movement beyond the natural range of movement of a joint may cause a vertebra to stay in that new (incorrect) position. It will then impinge on a nerve (by continuous pressure or stretching) over time.

Misalignments, traditionally called 'subluxations', are caused both by accidents and by the way we use our bodies in daily life. They occur during work, sport and childbirth, and from using inappropriate chairs and beds. Impingement upon the nerves can occur as they leave the spinal column or as they cross joints, altering the flow of impulses up and down the nerves, which interferes with the structural and functional integrity of the body.

The nerves come out of the spine through holes between the vertebrae (the intervertebral foramina). When there is a subluxation the shape of the relevant hole changes, thus altering the pressure on the nerve as it passes through and possibly causing impingement.

Subluxations cause a whole host of effects. There will be a change in the way the joint moves, and the point around which it moves. If the bone is fixed on one side, the other side tends to compensate by moving more, and will also move around the point that is fixed. If both sides are fixed, then the vertebrae above and below have to compensate, with the result that they become hypermobile (over-mobile).

If the nerve is squashed, the impulses passing down it build up, rather like water held behind a dam. Typical symptoms are pain, increased skin sensitivity, swelling, heat and muscle spasm, and overworking of any organ or gland which the nerve serves. In contrast, where the nerves are stretched there may be numbness or a sensation of pins and needles, loss of skin sensitivity, coldness,

What Can McTimoney Chiropractic Help?

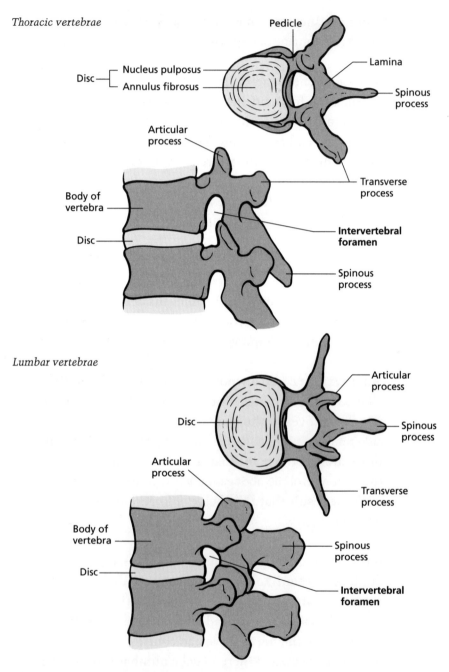

Thoracic vertebrae

Pedicle

Disc — [Nucleus pulposus
       Annulus fibrosus]

Lamina

Spinous process

Articular process

Transverse process

Body of vertebra

Intervertebral foramen

Disc

Spinous process

Lumbar vertebrae

Articular process

Disc

Spinous process

Articular process

Transverse process

Body of vertebra

Spinous process

Disc

Intervertebral foramen

The intervertebral foramina

muscle flaccidity and weakness and under-performance of any organ or gland supplied by that nerve.

Some nerves are very long, for example the sciatic nerve, which goes all the way from the lumbar area to the feet. This is why lumbar impingement can cause sciatic pain in the buttocks, hamstrings, calf muscles or feet, depending upon which of the nerve fibres are impinged.

Nerve fibres also pass through muscles and peripheral joints, and may become impinged there too by muscle spasm or peripheral joint subluxation. Sometimes there is even a combination of effects, where the nerve is impinged in two places, neither of which is sufficient to cause symptoms, but which together form a 'double crush'. Carpal tunnel syndrome and repetitive strain injury result from this sort of problem. The nerve is affected at both the neck and wrist, so that the arm muscles which are supplied by that nerve show no symptoms, but beyond the second 'crush', in the hand, you feel the pain and weakness.

Nerve Function

Nerve fibres are specific in their function and the messages they carry to and from the brain and muscle, joint, organ, area of skin, etc. – as set out in the Meric system.

There are motor nerves which deal with function, and sensory nerves which deal with sensation. Nerve fibres run in bundles, although there are several different pathways once the impulses reach the spine on the way to the brain. There is also a feedback system, so that if a nerve is impinged a collection of seemingly unrelated symptoms

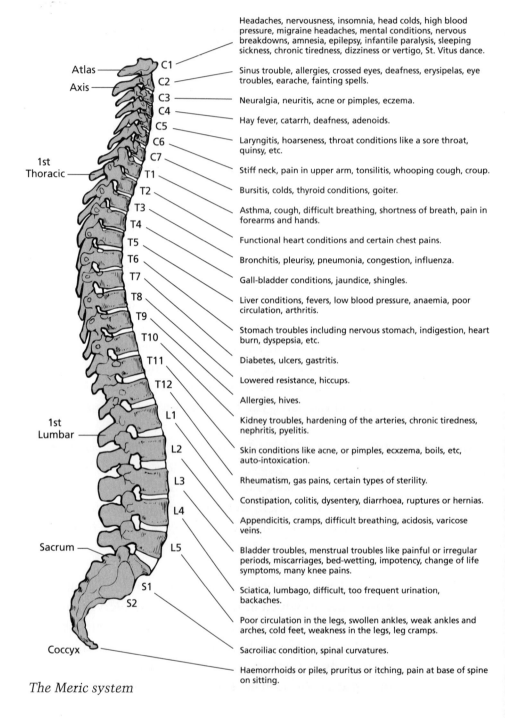

Headaches, nervousness, insomnia, head colds, high blood pressure, migraine headaches, mental conditions, nervous breakdowns, amnesia, epilepsy, infantile paralysis, sleeping sickness, chronic tiredness, dizziness or vertigo, St. Vitus dance.

Sinus trouble, allergies, crossed eyes, deafness, erysipelas, eye troubles, earache, fainting spells.

Neuralgia, neuritis, acne or pimples, eczema.

Hay fever, catarrh, deafness, adenoids.

Laryngitis, hoarseness, throat conditions like a sore throat, quinsy, etc.

Stiff neck, pain in upper arm, tonsilitis, whooping cough, croup.

Bursitis, colds, thyroid conditions, goiter.

Asthma, cough, difficult breathing, shortness of breath, pain in forearms and hands.

Functional heart conditions and certain chest pains.

Bronchitis, pleurisy, pneumonia, congestion, influenza.

Gall-bladder conditions, jaundice, shingles.

Liver conditions, fevers, low blood pressure, anaemia, poor circulation, arthritis.

Stomach troubles including nervous stomach, indigestion, heart burn, dyspepsia, etc.

Diabetes, ulcers, gastritis.

Lowered resistance, hiccups.

Allergies, hives.

Kidney troubles, hardening of the arteries, chronic tiredness, nephritis, pyelitis.

Skin conditions like acne, or pimples, ecxzema, boils, etc, auto-intoxication.

Rheumatism, gas pains, certain types of sterility.

Constipation, colitis, dysentery, diarrhoea, ruptures or hernias.

Appendicitis, cramps, difficult breathing, acidosis, varicose veins.

Bladder troubles, menstrual troubles like painful or irregular periods, miscarriages, bed-wetting, impotency, change of life symptoms, many knee pains.

Sciatica, lumbago, difficult, too frequent urination, backaches.

Poor circulation in the legs, swollen ankles, weak ankles and arches, cold feet, weakness in the legs, leg cramps.

Sacroiliac condition, spinal curvatures.

Haemorrhoids or piles, pruritus or itching, pain at base of spine on sitting.

The Meric system

(or just one type of symptom) may occur, depending upon which nerve fibres are impinged.

Associated Reactions

Frequently people suffer emotional and chemical reactions, as well as physical ones, to subluxation and nerve impingement. Sometimes there is one set of reactions to the main cause of impingement and then another set triggered by the compensation that the body makes in response to the first cause. Sometimes there are even several layers of compensation, which are built up as each level of tolerance is exceeded. As treatment progresses, these layers are gradually removed one by one, like peeling an onion. This is called 'retracing' and frequently occurs over a period of time, as in cases of recurring whiplash injuries. Old symptoms reappear temporarily, often as old memories, aches or malfunctions, and may seem like a relapse. You should discuss any reaction that arises like this with your chiropractor. Remember that it is a positive sign and is part of the healing process. Mostly, retracing manifests as a deep and satisfying sigh, as your body completes and sheds old, previously unfinished hurts, layer by layer.

Early Warning

When in pain we often grab the nearest painkiller instead of regarding it as a useful early warning sign. It is always far better to come for treatment while an injury is new and acute. This obviates the need for compensation and the storage of unfinished problems, which then become chronic. Acute injuries need far fewer treatments to put right than chronic.

What Can McTimoney Chiropractic Help?

Back Problems

Because of the popular notion that chiropractic is for back problems, it seems appropriate to start by looking at these. About 85 per cent of the population will experience back pain at least once during their lives: in the UK in 1993, 106 million days' sickness and invalidity benefit were paid out for back pain incapacities.[2]

The standard medical approach to back pain varies, depending upon the severity of the condition. Muscle relaxants, painkillers, rest and physiotherapy treatments such as traction, diathermy, ultrasound, hot packs and cold packs are sometimes used. However, these approaches have not always been found to be very helpful.[3]

If the problem doesn't improve or worsens, then surgery may be performed. In some cases surgery makes no difference or makes the pain even more intractable, and in others it does give long-term relief. However, many people who have had surgery report a recurrence of their symptoms within a few years and may return to the operating table. In contrast, studies such as the Manga Report (commissioned by the Government of Ontario, Canada) have found chiropractic care superior to medical care in terms of safety, scientific evidence of effectiveness, cost and patient satisfaction.

■ **A 42-year-old man had tingling in both his hands and both legs down to his toes. He also had a peptic ulcer and low back pain, which got worse when the ulcer flared up. His doctor** sent him to see a specialist, who was unable to see him for two months. In the mean time, he went to a McTimoney chiropractor. After the first treatment the tingling in his legs had gone. After eight treatments his back was fine, his ulcer had settled down and his fingers were improving. When he finally saw the neurosurgeon he was told that his body was 'healing itself' and there was no need to operate. ■

Apart from back pain and sciatica, chiropractic can help scoliosis, disc problems, sacro-iliac and hip problems and leg and foot pain.

Sciatic pain can affect both young and old:

■ A 17-year-old gymnast and dancer with severe sciatic pain was told by three doctors that as nothing showed on X-ray she should not worry – as she was young the condition would go away. It didn't. She became virtually paralysed down both legs. She then had a laminectomy (removal of the back part of one or more vertebrae to allow more space for the spinal cord) to treat two ruptured discs. She was not warned of any after-effects, but when she insisted on knowing, she was told she must restrict herself to walking and swimming, and would get calcification of the joints within two years. With great misgivings, she went to a McTimoney chiropractor. Next day, although she felt as if she had had a good work-out in the gym, she was pain-free with no neck, head or backache. She has since been trekking in the Himalayas and has qualified as a McTimoney chiropractor. Because of the nature of her work she has a treatment every two or three months and has developed no calcification. ■

Chiropractic can also help with the after-effects of accidents even in the elderly.

■ An active 76-year-old widow slipped when standing on a chair trying to open a jammed window in the bathroom. She fell backwards across the edge of the bath. When she came for McTimoney treatment, some six months after the accident, she was in continual, very severe pain and almost unable to walk. She was considering using a wheelchair. Chiropractic examination showed a right-hand curve in her thoraco-lumbar junction, which in the six months had become fairly immovable with adhesions and muscle spasm. Progress was slow at first, but after two months she was able to move more freely. A month later this delightful elderly lady, whose favourite activity was ballroom dancing, came in to say she had done two waltzes and a fox-trot! In all over a period of nearly four months and 23 treatments, she made a full recovery. ■

Such a large number of treatments is unusual, and may have been necessary because of her age. The next case was left equally long before treatment; if treated sooner it may not have been so severe:

■ A 36-year-old mechanic wrenched the middle of his back while lifting an engine out of a car. He was off work for six months with an excruciating knife-like pain on the left of his mid-spine. When he came for McTimoney treatment he had tried all the conventional treatment routes, and was very distressed that at his fairly young age he might be an invalid for the rest of his life, especially as he had three young children to support. This previously fit man used to work out at a gym three nights a week; now he had lost three stone (42 lb) in weight and was emaciated. The weight loss was consistent with the area of the spine from which the pain came, because the nerves from that area also serve the stomach. Every meal he had eaten for the past six months had passed through his system almost undigested, accounting for the weight loss.

The chiropractic findings included two jammed mid-thoracic vertebrae and a lot of local muscle spasm. After the first treatment, he gained 7 lb in weight and the pain was reduced by half. When he came for the second treatment a week later he had gained a stone (14 lb) in weight and was virtually pain-free. After the third treatment he went back to work totally recovered. ■

Headaches, Migraines and Facial Problems

The head and neck are also areas that commonly cause debilitating problems. Headaches have numerous causes: they can be mental (as in the case of those suffering high stress levels), physical (as in muscle spasm and/or subluxated vertebrae in the neck) or chemical, resulting from the use of drugs or alcohol, volatile oils and strong smells, sinus infections, or from visual, dental or ear problems. Millions of pounds a year are spent on painkillers which remove the symptoms, but not the cause, and the long-term ingestion of such drugs can cause side-effects. One study of 6,000 long-term headaches revealed that neck injury (whiplash, falls) was the most important factor causing headaches and should be suspected in every non-specific case of headache.[4] Migraine can involve both a severe headache and a visual disturbance.

Passing through the neck are all the blood and nerve supplies between the body and brain, as well as the muscles to hold up and balance the heaviest body part against gravity. Considering all this, *and* that the neck still has to be flexible in all ranges of movement, it is amazing that it doesn't malfunction more often! Headaches frequently arise from tense neck muscles impinging the sub-occipital nerve as it passes over the ridge in the occipital bone on either side at the top of the neck. This is a recurrent occupational problem with desk workers and musicians (*see the case histories in the section on Sport and Work Injuries, page 91*), particularly if there is a constant twist to one side when reading a manuscript to type or when holding a violin. Headache also occurs as a result of compensation: for example, the head is poked forward, tensing the neck muscles, when the pelvis is tipped backward by a seat that slopes back, as when lounging on a sofa to watch TV.

■ **A 12-year-old schoolgirl who usually enjoyed good health was taken to her doctor with an extremely severe headache – so bad that her parents feared she had meningitis. Her doctor diagnosed migraine and gave her medication. Forty-eight hours later, and after a good sleep, she felt better and was able to go to school. Three weeks later she became ill again with the same type of headache. The medication was repeated and again she recovered. This pattern was repeated twice more, so her parents decided to try McTimoney chiropractic. After two treatments she is headache-free. ■**

Headaches can also occur as a result of old, unresolved childhood injuries:

■ **A woman had been suffering headaches of varying severity several times a week, with migraines two or three times a year, for several years. With the onset of the menopause these became a daily occurrence, and she woke with a bad headache in the small hours every morning. The headache would persist all day until 5 p.m., when she would begin to yawn. It would then begin to lift and by 11 p.m. she would be pain-free, only to start suffering again between 1 and 2 a.m. She also had Irritable Bowel Syndrome.**

The Essentials of McTimoney Chiropractic

She had tried acupuncture, homoeopathy, relaxation exercises, hypnotherapy, zero-balancing and osteopathy, massage and yoga. She had explored her past emotional problems with a psychiatrist, tried colour therapy, diet changes and fasting. They all helped to some extent, but ultimately provided no major benefit or insight.

After a frightening course of Lithium prescribed by a migraine specialist, on a recommendation but without any real hope, she contacted a McTimoney chiropractor. Because of her previous experiences she was unprepared for the immediate feeling of lightness and freedom following the treatment, and was surprised at how holistic, gentle and painless it was. The chiropractor explained the connection between Irritable Bowel Syndrome and headaches, and how she could help herself by making changes to her lifestyle and diet. A week after her first treatment she had six pain-free days, which in her words 'made history' for her. After having had headaches for 35 years, in six months she has had a 75 per cent reduction in severity and 40 per cent reduction in frequency – the IBS/migraine link is still there, but muted. Now, waking at 2 a.m. with a migraine is a rare event, and when she does, she knows the cause. She can work with this reduced headache and no longer dreads having to bend down or being in an airless office or near unshuttered windows on a bright day. ■

Because McTimoney chiropractic adjusts the bones of the face and jaw it can be extremely effective in reducing pain in these areas. Trigeminal neuralgia is an extremely painful form of facial neuralgia, normally quite difficult to treat.

■ A 28-year-old woman suffered excruciating facial pain for three years, and after five consecutive nights when she could

What Can McTimoney Chiropractic Help?

neither sleep nor lie horizontally she went to her doctor. She was prescribed Ibuprofen and was told to see a dentist. She subsequently tried every painkiller she could buy, but none touched the pain. The dentist diagnosed the problem as trigeminal neuralgia and prescribed Tergatol, which at least enabled her to sleep. However it also produced side-effects of paranoia, nausea, rash and drowsiness, and even affected her eyesight, which became worse with repeated use. She was still losing hours of sleep.

She came to the conclusion that modern medicine had nothing more to offer and went to see a McTimoney chiropractor. Since her first treatment, she has only had three mild attacks in three months – all treatable with over-the-counter painkillers. ■

■ A secretary aged 35 was unable to close her jaw so that her teeth met properly on one side of her mouth. Before embarking on major dental work (involving crowning all the teeth on one side of her mouth to correct her bite) she decided to try chiropractic. She was astonished to find that after one treatment her bite had returned to normal, and she has had no further problems. ■

Shoulders, Arms and Hands

After the neck and back, the most common problems seen by chiropractors occur in the shoulders. The nerve supply to the shoulders, arms and hands (the brachial plexus) passes through the muscles of the middle and lower neck and upper back. This means that any arm, wrist or hand problems can be affected by neck misalignments, hence the particular focus put upon the area by all chiropractors.

McTimoney chiropractors always also consider the whole body alignment as well as the actual site of the pain, in case the neck misalignment is a result of compensation.

■ **A 40-year-old businessman who was also a semi-professional tennis player had suffered for two and a half years from shoulder pain. When he finally saw a McTimoney chiropractor he was asked if anyone had checked his pelvis. No one had. After one treatment, he experienced some improvement, and after five, he was pain-free and back on the tennis court. ■**

■ **Another businessman slipped down a frosty stone staircase. He got up, flustered, and subsequently felt pins and needles in his back which he ignored. Months later, sitting at the piano, he felt an 'electric shock' shoot through his neck, shoulder and arm. His arm became continuously painful and – in varying degrees at various times – he lost control of it and the ability to use it. A severe pain then developed in his neck, and his head felt too heavy to hold up. He got to the point where even writing was extremely uncomfortable. Any sport was out of the question.**

On visiting a McTimoney chiropractor he was impressed by the explanation of chiropractic he was given, but was uneasy when he had no immediate response – although the chiropractor had warned him this might happen. However, after a couple more treatments his condition improved dramatically, and he began playing golf and tennis again. ■

Our hands can often take a battering, for instance when they break a fall for us, as happened to the following woman:

What Can McTimoney Chiropractic Help?

■ A 55-year-old housewife fell heavily on a gravel path, hitting her right cheekbone, shoulder, ribs, hip and knee. Hardest of all she hit her right hand, which was under her body as she fell. It was extremely painful and swollen, and she took arnica to alleviate the bruising and shock. She was unable to use her hand, but since no bones were broken she didn't go to her doctor. After four weeks, however, it still hadn't healed and, as she feared it never would, she went to a McTimoney chiropractor. Two treatments later her hand had recovered fully; the pain had gone and she had full mobility. ■

Often people go to a chiropractor because they learn from the experience of friends and relatives of the many problems that can be helped by it:

■ An 85-year-old man came to a McTimoney chiropractor with his wife, who was suffering from back and shoulder pain. He watched her being treated, and was delighted when, after four treatments, she was free from pain. He then asked if chiropractic could help his Dupuytren's contracture (a progressive hand condition in which the fingers and sometimes the thumb curl over so that the hand cannot be opened sufficiently to grasp objects). The condition affected both his hands. After only two treatments he could open his hands fully, and the problem has not thus far recurred. ■

Gynaecological Problems

When a patient comes to see a chiropractor for the first time, a very full history is taken of *all* their symptoms, not just the ones that caused them to seek treatment in the first place. This thoroughness often pays dividends. Since there is both a muscular and a nervous link between the uterus and the spine, adjustment can lead to easier menstruation, with periods becoming more regular and less painful. In one study of 122 dysmenorrhea sufferers, most had low back problems and spinal displacement.[5]

Pregnancy, especially in the later stages, causes a change in the body's centre of gravity. This can create an increased curve in the lumbar spine, and many women suffer back pain at this time. Gentle and well-supported treatment by McTimoney chiropractic can ease this problem.

It can also be very helpful to have treatment after giving birth. The birth process necessitates a softening of the ligaments in the pelvic area. If there is any difficulty with presentation or birth, the mother's pelvic bones may not realign themselves correctly afterwards; chiropractic can help to realign any misalignments occurring in this way.

Since most members of the public associate chiropractic primarily with back pain, it comes as a surprise that apparently non-physical problems can be treated too. There are strong links between the spine, the nerves and the hormonal system. Postnatal depression may sound an unlikely candidate for chiropractic treatment, yet the following case is typical:

■ **A mother arrived in a state of near collapse and in floods of tears at a McTimoney clinic, carrying her 10-day-old daughter. Three days later the chiropractor received a card from her saying 'I can never thank you enough for what you did for me, it was like a miracle. I still get a little weepy, no doubt due to lack of sleep, but I no longer feel "strange" – it's wonderful.'** ■

Few women make a connection between the type of contraceptive method they use and back pain. But pain can refer back to the spine or back from a badly fitting IUD or coil, in which case other forms of contraception may be more appropriate. Many women are also affected by back pain following gynaecological operations such as hysterectomy and D & C. This may be due to the way the operations are performed, which puts a lot of stress on the lower back. In these cases, chiropractic can help. (If a woman already has back problems, it's certainly worth informing the surgeon before surgery, because then he or she will usually arrange for her back to be supported by extra pillows during the operation.)

Other Common Problems

Chiropractic can improve your general health because it directly boosts the immune system. The science of psychoneuroimmunology shows that the nervous system communicates directly with the immune system and the endocrine system. Thus chiropractic can also improve the body's self-healing powers.

■ **A 59-year-old nursing auxiliary, already being treated for diabetes, attended a McTimoney chiropractic clinic suffering from pain in the neck, shoulders, low back, both thighs and ankles. She had been diagnosed by her doctor as having rheumatoid arthritis, although there was no joint swelling or raised ESR (a test commonly carried out in diagnosing arthritis). After one McTimoney treatment she had two pain-free days, but then the symptoms returned. After the second treatment she had a strong reaction and was in severe pain for 48 hours, followed by feeling much freer. After 12 treatments over the course of a year, all her pain had gone**

completely. At a subsequent visit to the endocrinologist who was treating her insulin-dependent diabetes, she was advised that her blood sugar was so well under control that she could now stop the injections and control her condition with diet and tablets alone. ■

Stress and blood pressure problems can also respond to the realignment of subluxations, because all misalignments sap the body's available energy, strength and healing power, causing low energy levels and depression, or that constant feeling of tiredness well known to many women, particularly those running both a career and a family. (Of course, men are not exempt either!)

Being ill enough to stay in bed beyond the normal length of time required for proper sleep (particularly if accompanied by a fever and/or aches and pains, as can occur with flu, for example) means that the body may need a check-up. It is also very important to check with your chiropractor if your bed is too hard or too soft (remember, even though the bed is right for your partner it may not be right for you!).

Other conditions which may not seem obvious candidates for chiropractic are ear infections, tinnitus and deafness, and even some eye problems. The second cervical (neck) vertebra affects the nerve supply to the middle ear, and that vertebra can be misaligned because it is compensating for a problem lower down the spine.

Problems in the area of the head are often due to cranial (skull) misalignment. The bones of the head fit very closely together with tongue-and-groove or bevel joints, interlocked like gear cogs. Misalignment of one bone will cause torsion

What Can McTimoney Chiropractic Help?

on all the others and squeeze the cranial nerves as they pass between one bone and another within the head cavity or as they leave the skull. The meninges (the three layers of protective fibrous material protecting the brain and spinal cord) are only attached to the inside of the cranium, the top two neck vertebrae, and then there are no further attachments until the lowest back vertebrae. Because the meninges are somewhat inelastic, a misaligned pelvis will pull on the meninges, and this pull will extend up to the top of the spine and the cranium. This means that frequently both the cranium and pelvis are similarly misaligned. Only a whole-body treatment will take this into account.

There are many examples of this. One woman returned for a second treatment for her back, delighted to announce her tinnitus was cured; another found relief for lifelong deafness in her left ear. One McTimoney practitioner has helped five people to recover their hearing, and one 50-year-old woman is now breathing properly through her nose for the first time in her life.

■ **A 30-year-old housewife was blind in one eye and was waiting for an operation to have it removed and a glass one fitted. In the mean time she developed low back pain and came for chiropractic treatment. After one treatment she realized she could see with both eyes again. She needed three further treatments for her back, but 26 years on she retains the sight in both eyes!** ■

Although this is a real case history (as are all the others given here), it would not be wise to bank on this kind of result *every* time! It depends very much on individual conditions.

Sport and Work Injuries

Competitive sports usually cause us to stretch and test our bodies more than normal, and are often the cause of injuries. At the risk of repetition, it is always best to come for chiropractic treatment as soon as you notice a problem, however slight. Good alignment makes for economy of body use, faster reactions and greater control. Many sports require one-sided body use, and a McTimoney chiropractor can advise you on how to avoid the problems that may arise from building up muscles more on one side of the body than the other (*see also Chapter 6*).

Workplaces are often poorly arranged from the body's point of view, and here again chiropractic ergonomic advice is helpful. I quote from a practitioner asked to advise the managers of a factory on how to protect their workers from back pain and other problems such as repetitive strain injury (RSI):

There were 40 men and women between 20 and 40 years of age. On examination not one employee was totally free from pain; ranging from headaches, neck and shoulder pain, elbow pain, carpal tunnel syndrome, mid-back and lower back pain, rib pain, to pins and needles in the legs and knee pain.

Over a period of six weeks this workforce were treated once a week as necessary. Some of them only needed two treatments. They were all doing the same job and nobody had any time off work. Preventative advice was given to help the workers avoid a return of their problems. There was at least a 90 per cent success rate.

The performing arts can also put great strains on the body, whether through playing musical instruments or the heavy demands of dancing.

■ **A 16-year-old violinist suffered headaches when playing. She also had left knee pain, and both foot arches were dropped, causing difficulty with walking for more than 10 minutes. Physiotherapy was tried but didn't help. However, after six sessions with a McTimoney chiropractor all her symptoms were gone and have not returned over the past three years.** ■

■ **A 35-year-old dancer and choreographer with the Royal Ballet experienced a sudden onset of very severe low back pain one morning. He had had no previous back problems and was otherwise in good health. He went for chiropractic treatment as soon as possible. He was amazed that it did not hurt and was delighted to find that he was able to dance the very next day. It was explained to him that the reason he recovered so quickly was that his muscle tone was excellent and that he had sought treatment without delay.** ■

Nurses are frequent sufferers of back problems, due to the nature of their work.

■ **A 32-year-old hospital nurse had been suffering from low back pain for several years. The pain had become so severe that she had to give up her job. She came for chiropractic treatment and was astonished at how quickly she felt the benefits. By the second treatment she was thinking about returning to nursing. Over a period of five weeks she received six treatments and advice on lifting properly. A few months later she returned to nursing and had no further problems.**

Three years after this she suffered a fall, injuring her shoulder. Realizing that chiropractic copes with much more than just back pain, she returned for treatment and her shoulder problem was solved.

This nurse's mother, having witnessed her daughter's successful treatment, decided to see a chiropractor for help with the migraines she had suffered from for 29 years. After just three treatments she had no further migraines, and has not suffered another in the past five years. The only thing that saddens her is that she did not seek McTimoney treatment sooner. ∎

As this chapter shows, there is a very wide range of conditions that can be treated when a whole-body treatment is carried out at every visit. The importance of immediate treatment (rather than waiting and hoping symptoms will go away) is clearly demonstrated by the case histories in this chapter.

The case histories in this chapter were supplied by experienced McTimoney chiropractors Susan Cartlidge, Dana Green, Alison Gordon-Creed, Stan Harding, Barbara Minter and Christina Cunliffe. A high proportion of practitioners have become chiropractors because of the chiropractic treatment and help they themselves have received, and while some of the case histories may seem spectacular, they are by no means unusual. It is worth remembering that while the rule of thumb for most manipulative techniques is that a month's treatment is required for every year that the problem has existed, the average number of treatments needed per McTimoney patient is between four and six.

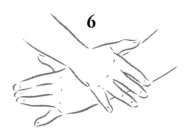

6

SELF-HELP

When you take a course of McTimoney treatments your practitioner is very likely to encourage you to practise self-help. This usually begins between treatments to back up your chiropractic sessions, and continues afterwards with maintenance and prevention techniques.

Self-help makes good sense when you realize that, although you may see your chiropractor once a week while undergoing treatment, you actually live with your body 24 hours a day: this makes you an expert on it. Successful self-help depends on personal responsibility and is part and parcel of wellness behaviour. It depends upon adequate knowledge of the possibilities and options open to you, and then making the choice to help yourself. In this chapter you will find discussions on wellness and illness behaviours, understanding your body's reactions through observation and balancing body use, and other factors that can affect your posture and cause aches and pains.

Responsibility for yourself in a chiropractic situation might sound terribly serious, complicated and hard work; actually it simply implies a few moments' thought and awareness about sensible, balanced care and consideration for your body, in how you use it, exercise it, feed it and look after it in general. We are so obsessed with success at work and the need to achieve more, better, faster and longer that we forget the second part of the old adage 'a healthy mind *in a healthy body'*. We ignore our bodies all week while we earn our living, and then expect them to perform miracles on the tennis court or golf course at the weekend. Many of us pay scant attention to what happens to us below the neck until it shouts for attention, and then we go to an expert to get it mended as if it were a car or a washing machine, and without expecting to take part in or be responsible for the repairs.

To some extent this attitude is fostered by the medical profession which expects you to 'leave it to the doctor who knows best', and where diagnosis dictates treatment. By and large, medical treatment is directed at suppressing symptoms which means you can continue on in your own sweet way – until the symptoms return, when the treatment or prescription will probably be repeated. Rarely does the medical profession have the time or resources to look at preventative methods. At best, if you require phys-iotherapy you will probably be given six sessions. Appointment times do not allow for anything further, and the only responsibility you have if a cure is not effected by then is to believe that nothing more can be done and that you will 'have to learn to live with it'. Don't believe it. It usually means they don't know what else to do or suggest to help you.

The Importance of Attitude

Attitude – your state of mind and what you believe – is vitally important in healing. There is a well-recognized behaviour pattern associated with illness. It is characterized by:

- waiting – for an appointment, for others to help you or do something for or to you, or even dependency physically and emotionally, to the extent of controlling those caring for you;

- poor sleeping, malaise, low energy or low stamina, inertia;

- depression, lack of self esteem, institutionalization, obsession, despair, giving up trying;

- feeling weak and incapable about, yet absorbed by, your problem, which you rehearse endlessly, boring everyone around you.

Of course we all suffer some of these behaviour patterns occasionally, but as ways of being, they are typical of chronically ill people who do not know how to help themselves.

Wellness behaviour is quite the opposite. Even if not entirely fit, you are full of plans for what you can already do, what you will do soon and what the future holds for you. You see lots of possibilities, you give out a feeling of initiative, energy and enthusiasm, and can't wait to get started. You ask lots of questions about how you can help yourself, and while you don't ignore your problems, you give them only the attention they deserve, doing what you can and then trusting your body's innate healing process. You are far more interested in everyone else than in your own problems, and may even think in terms of how you can help them too.

Avoiding Surgery

A frequent reason for seeing a chiropractor is to avoid surgery – which often seems the only medical solution left to spinal and joint problems. Surgery is salvage work. Once you have something surgically cut or removed, it can't be replaced or returned to its original state: there will always be inelastic scar tissue to cope with. Surgery should therefore only be considered as a last resort, and as a surgeon himself has put it, 'surgeons often have a reputation for being knife-happy, insensitive and crude ... The surgeon should be right at the bottom of the filter.[1] There is often much work that can be done by you before that turning to [that] "last resort".'

Doing what you can to help yourself may include learning a small amount of simple basic postures and body use, anatomy or physiology, so that you understand the relevance of the exercises that your chiropractor asks you to do. The chiropractor works with you rather than imposing upon you, and the more you can bring to the partnership in the form of doing agreed exercises and following other preventative advice, the better you will maintain good health.

The Essentials of McTimoney Chiropractic

Ideally there will be a partnership between you and your chiropractor to realign your body. He or she will then motivate and teach you the physical tools to keep it fit, so that ultimately, all you will need is the occasional check-up.

Between treatments you may be asked to observe your posture and body use. It is useful here to understand the difference between the sort of posture you see illustrated in books on posture, showing a plumb-line passing through various areas of the body – a two-dimensional diagram – and actual body use, which is three-dimensional.

Posture

On a diagram, seen from the front, the vertical line passes between the eyebrows, through the nose, the chin, the sternal notch (the dip between your collarbones), and through your tummy button, then drops to the floor equidistant from the knees and ankles. At the back, the same line passes through the centre of the head and neck, between the shoulder blades, following the line of the spine through the buttocks and on down to the floor.

Horizontal lines should pass across the eyebrows, the earlobes should be level, as should the shoulders, elbows, nipples, hips, knees and ankles. There should be equal spaces between the elbows and the body, and the hands and feet should be turned so that the thumbs and big toes all face forward. The knees should face forward rather than towards or away from each other.

Seen from the side, the vertical line should pass through the top centre of the head, the ear hole and the middle of

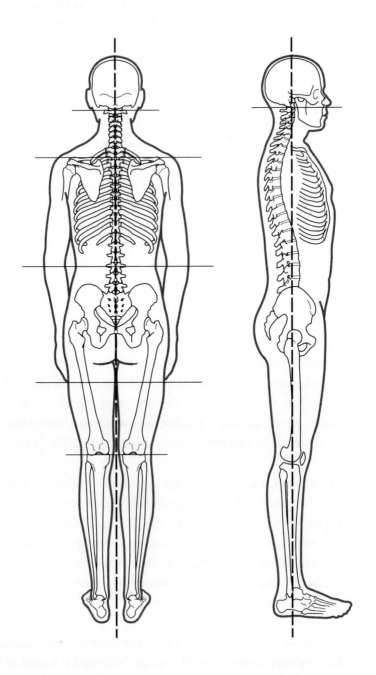

the shoulder. The line should then pass just behind the head of the thigh bone, through the centre of the knee and just in front of the ankle. Horizontally, the nostrils should be level with the centre of the ear.

These, of course, are rather rigid ideals of perfection which do not take account of real life, with the effect that if you aim to follow them without any understanding, you may tend to become rigid too. Textbooks forget that the body is three-dimensional and built for movement. How you use your body actually determines its posture, in that frequent use in a specific way builds some muscles more than others. Continued one-sided use, as in the case of golfers or hod-carriers, means that habits are formed which then become automatic and subconscious, and your posture is set.

It is also well known that specific postures predispose people to certain diseases. Mostly this occurs when an area becomes squashed, for example digestive problems often occur in people who slump. The converse is true, too: poor posture often follows stressed use, as in asthmatics who often have a high breast bone and barrel chest. The process begins with acute physical symptoms, then compensation or adaptation follows to handle the physical stress caused by these symptoms, then further adaptations follow to handle the adaptations as they become fatigued and chronic. Finally the body tries to stabilize over-mobile joints by growing arthritic spurs, or the organs squashed by faulty posture and poor nerve supply constantly malfunction, leading to a predisposition to disease.

Regretfully, children frequently copy the posture of the most significant adults in their lives, which is why some diseases seem to run in families even when they are apparently not inherited via genes.

If you wish to check your own posture, you may find it useful to string up a plumb line in front of a long mirror to train your vision. Stand in front of it with your eyes closed and move about until you feel you are standing absolutely straight. Without moving your body, open your eyes and look. You will be surprised. What you see is unlikely to be as straight as it feels. It will be a picture of your subconscious adaptations, which only feel right because you are used to them.

Self-observation

It is even more important to observe *how* you use your body in daily life. Although you may have a preference – that is, you will be right- or left-handed – your body is built to be used equally on both sides. Obviously, where accuracy is important (as when cutting bread, playing darts or writing) you should use your dominant hand and eye, but where it is not (putting on a coat, shaving or cleaning your teeth, vacuuming the floor), experiment with using both hands or both sides of your body. At first this will feel strange and uncoordinated, but it will become natural with practice.

There are times when swapping sides is impossible because of tradition, such as mounting a horse from the left, or because the machine or implement you are using is built in a certain way, as with scissors, a flute or violin, golf clubs or tennis racquet, the position of a VDU mouse, or the direction of a production line. You can still help yourself. When you have finished the job, reduce the biased use: have a good long stretch (10–20 seconds) in the opposite direction, mirror-imaging what the occupation forced you to do, and then return to a normal, central, equally weighted standing position.

Standing

People spend a lot of their time standing, yet rarely do they stand with their weight equally on both feet. When they sit they often cross their legs. Standing with your weight unevenly distributed causes a hip tilt and torque (twist) to maintain balance. One side goes up and back, the other goes down and forward. The problem is not that you do this, but that you always do it one way 'because it's easier'. You will probably catch yourself doing this when you are waiting for something, or are preoccupied as when waiting for a bus, at a party, doing the washing up, shaving, waiting for that call back and so on.

The first self-help step here is to observe yourself and others. This will not only train your eye and awareness, but also make you realize how common the fault is. Compare the posture of a toddler with that of an older person. The toddler moves freely and uses his or her body efficiently. The older person usually has to contend with a collection of unsolved postural problems and compensations. Only when you become conscious of what you are doing, and that *you* are doing it, can you have the choice whether or not to do something about it and change to the other side. Remember the other side only feels odd because it's unpractised and inexperienced. You will not remember to change sides every time at first, but every time you do remember, change sides

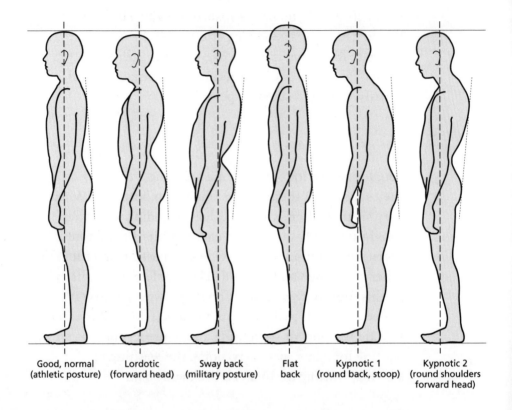

| Good, normal (athletic posture) | Lordotic (forward head) | Sway back (military posture) | Flat back | Kypnotic 1 (round back, stoop) | Kypnotic 2 (round shoulders forward head) |

until it doesn't matter on which side you perform a particular action.

The rule is 1: Observe, 2: Make a conscious choice, 3: Counteract.

Compensation

Apart from obvious accidents, falls or operations, compensation is a common cause of one or more subluxations. An example of this might be someone with a foot problem (such as a dropped arch, corns or a twisted ankle). Putting weight on that foot will cause pain, so you either put your weight on the other leg, or you change the angle at which you put your foot down, which in turn affects the angle at the knee joint. Either of these may cause the hip joints to be unevenly affected, and with them alter the alignment of the pelvis, either tilting it or torquing one side against the other. An uneven pelvis means that the spine is no longer vertical, and somewhere along its length it has to bend in order for your eyes to be level. If the compensating bend is in the low back you will have low back pain, if in the mid back, you will have pain in that area. If it is in the shoulders, neck or just under the head, that is where the pain will be. You may even get headaches because the shoulders are not level, causing an uneven pull of the neck muscles on the back of the head. Thus from a foot problem we arrive at a headache!

There may of course be any combination of compensations, but pain is always felt in the last area to compensate and become fatigued. Since the spine is less mobile in the areas held by the pelvis, ribs and head, the bits in between, the low back and neck, are freer to move and consequently are the most common areas where compensation and pain occur.

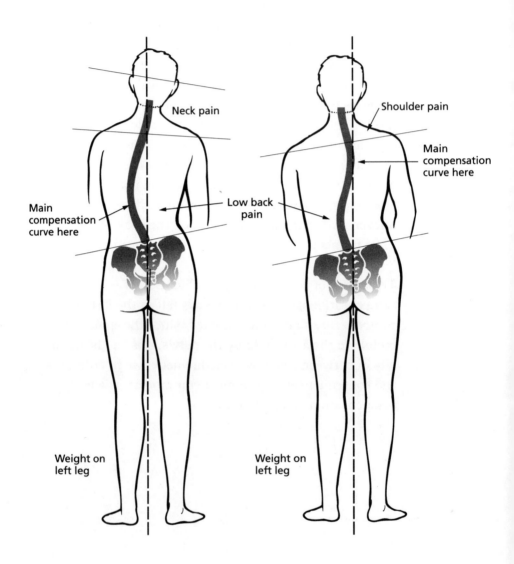

Neck pain

Shoulder pain

Main
compensation
curve here

Main
compensation
curve here

Low back
pain

Weight on
left leg

Weight on
left leg

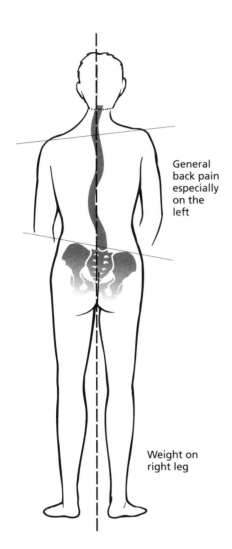

General
back pain
especially
on the
left

Weight on
right leg

Other Causes of Postural Problems: Furniture and Fashion

Your posture may also be affected by outside forces such as wearing high heels, seating – the type of chairs, car, plane and coach seats you have to use – and your bed. Worse still, in the smaller car and van range the foot pedals are often offset because of lack of room, so that in order to drive you end up with a constant slight twist on the spine. This twist also occurs if you spend hours watching a TV that is not directly in front of you. The placing of work stations and office furniture can cause similar problems. The body can only tolerate these twists for a short while before muscle fatigue sets in: constant repetition, or constantly holding the body in one position, can bring you to the limit of tolerance so that stiffness and pain occur. This poor body use may become an habitual posture to which other parts of your body will have to accommodate or compensate. You can and should counteract this by stretching in the opposite direction. This undoes the knots and brings your body back to the centre of its range of motion.

Beds

Beds are often blamed for back problems because they are too soft. There is a fallacy that the harder the bed, the better it is for your back. What you actually need is one that allows you to keep your spine in alignment when you lie on your back, but with enough give to allow for your shoulders and hips when lying on your side. When you buy a mattress, take someone with you who can check that your spine is straight and parallel to the floor when you lie on it sideways, and do not assume that what is right for you is also correct for your partner. The same

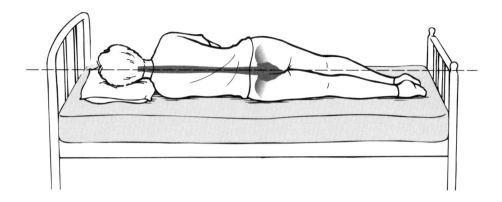

goes for pillows – you need enough bulk to fill up the space between your head and shoulders when you lie on your side, yet still be able to keep some neck curve when you lie on your back.

High Heels

Wearing high heels may look elegant and make you appear taller, but they drastically affect posture. They throw your weight on to the front of your foot so that your toes are thrust into the front of the shoe. Your calf muscles are kept constantly short, and you can only stand upright by locking your knees back and bending back from the waist. This not only contracts the lumbar muscles but also throws your shoulders back, so that you have to poke your head (or at least your chin) forward in order to look straight ahead. No wonder people complain 'my feet are killing me' and kick off their shoes the minute they get home! Even better would be to make a point of stretching 'mirror image' to undo those poor calf, back and neck muscles.

Stand on your toes on the edge of a step, facing the top of the staircase. While steadying yourself, let your heels sink down below the level of your toes for 10 seconds.

Next, come away from the staircase and flop forward from the waist (knees straight but not locked back) to undo the lumbar muscles. Come up again slowly, lengthening the neck by straightening it as if pulled up by a string at the top of your head; finally, let the head flop forward on to your chest for a few seconds.

Seating

Chairs, car seats, bus and plane seats are a constant problem. They are designed for lounging in, for the average person (and very few of us are average in all dimensions) or perhaps as a design feature in a house or car, or for easy stacking in a hall or auditorium. They are not usually made to maintain good posture or to work in. Most have backward-sloping seats with or without sloping backs, and they may also be bucket-shaped, all of which will either maintain the problem you already have or make it worse.

Just as high heels throw your weight forward, these backward-sloping seats throw it backward, and with it your pelvis. In order to sit upright, with each vertebra sitting easily and naturally on the one below, you have to sit on the front of the chair, holding the pelvis forward against gravity and the slope of the seat by maintaining constantly contracted muscles. Car seats often have a bulging cushion in the lumbar area and a head rest. Neither of these may be correctly positioned for you, and while the head rest is often movable, the lumbar bulge rarely is.

The Essentials of McTimoney Chiropractic

Postural Aids

If the world seems expressly designed to exacerbate your postural problem, what can you do about it? One solution comes in the form of postural aids. There are many kinds: cushions, wedges, blow-up versions of these, piano cups, or blocks, boards and specially designed chairs and mattresses. All are good in some situations, all have disadvantages. The first three are something extra to have to carry about, can be expensive and can also very easily be left behind by mistake. Cups and blocks to put under chair legs are bulky, as are bed boards. Specially designed chairs and mattresses are expensive, but they do mean that you can have exactly what you want at home: a visit to a specialist back care shop will help you find what you need. When away from home, unfortunately, you have to take pot luck, and do mirror image stretches if necessary. Meanwhile, before you spend money it's a good idea to discuss the matter thoroughly with your chiropractor to find out exactly what you need and where, by experimenting with a folded or rolled hand-towel or a 1-metre square piece of bubble pack – which is cheap, light to carry, draft- and water-proof, and can be turned into an instant cushion anywhere.

Lifting

Lifting weights inappropriately may have been the original cause of your back problem. As part of your rehabilitation, your chiropractor will teach you how to lift with minimum injury to yourself, or may suggest you study the guidelines set out for nurses if your normal routine includes caring for an elderly relative or looking after young children. If lifting is part of your work you should be trained by your firm as part of their health and safety policy.

In general the three cardinal points when it comes to lifting are:

1 Divide the weight if you can (use several shopping bags rather than putting it all in one big box).

2 Keep the weight close to you.

3 Keep your back straight, bend your knees and lift by straightening them.

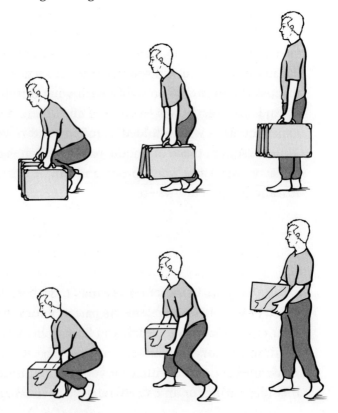

Stress

All of us react to too much stress physically as well as mentally. Some of us clench our buttocks, others grind their teeth, yet others get stiff necks or their shoulders rise up round their ears. The body acts out our feelings and always tells the truth whether you like it or not, and no matter how much you try to hide it.

The media mostly concentrate on the negative aspects of stress. Actually we all need a certain amount of stimulation and stress. What's called for is the appropriate amount of stress, a balance between the task we are engaged in and how we feel about it: stress is not in things out there, it is in us – in how we react to events.

On the positive side it is very useful to be aware of your state of mind or attitude, your pulse rate and all the other arbiters of stress that occur when you perform at your peak in any competitive situation. This same state is entirely inappropriate, however, when you wish to rest and recuperate. Knowing your own signs and signals – 'what makes you tick' or 'gets you going' – is good stress management.

On the negative side, to ignore or not to recognize the signs causes a stress buildup. Our bodies act out that which our minds can't handle, as a direct response to a nervous system over-stimulated by adrenaline, and we get similar effects to those of nerve impingement even though a different part of the nervous system is involved. Too much stress leads to back ache, neck ache, headache, and abdominal aches and pains as the digestive system is affected, and prolonged stress will lower the immune response or our tolerance for noxious substances. The symptoms you get depend upon which is your weakest area – this area will be affected first.

It may therefore be useful, if you recognize a recurring pain, to ask yourself what other stresses coincide with it each time it occurs. They are usually emotional. You may get a stiff back at times when you feel a lack of support in your life, or you may have a stiff neck when having to do something you do not really wish to do. There is a clash between the logical brain and the emotional body, which meet at the neck – which is pulled in two ways at once and so jams. Often if you know why a pain is there it is less frightening, you are more in control and, if you can resolve the situation, the muscle spasm causing the misalignments goes – as does the pain.

If you have difficulty in handling your stress alone it might be appropriate to have counselling therapy at the same time as chiropractic (as long as each practitioner is informed about the other).

Diet and Weight

Although not part of chiropractic *per se*, nutrition and optimum weight are of vital importance to general health and definitely form part of any self-help, maintenance and prevention regime. Just as impingement of the nervous system can affect your digestion and overall health, so your digestion can affect what nutrition is available for growth, repair, storage, resistance to stress and disease.

Being overweight is a constant strain on the body, over-stressing the knee joints, inhibiting freedom of movement and slowing down blood and lymph flow, and with it the distribution of the appropriate nutrition and removal of waste products from the muscles and joints.

From a structural point of view, a protruding belly and weak abdominal muscles add to the stress on the back muscles, which have to work hard to hold your front ribs up and out of your pelvis. This causes lumbar hyper-lordosis (an increased curve in the lower back), which upsets the centre of gravity in the same way as wearing high heels does. The vertebrae in the low back become tipped back and crowded, causing impingement and adding one-sided pressure on the discs, which can then herniate or prolapse easily. Your McTimoney chiropractor will be pleased to discuss a reasonable diet with you and may suggest a suitable sport or exercises that you can do at home or at your local gym.

Exercise and Sport

Attempting to lessen stress by playing sport vigorously may help temporarily, but it is often a form of 'symptom swatting' so that you don't feel the pain or play through it. It may divert and distract you, but the pain will return unless the stress itself is dealt with. Eventually you will need to resolve the reason for your tension and adverse reaction to circumstances. You will need to find a balance.

There is no doubt that using Yoga, Alexander and Feldenkrais techniques, going to the gym or swimming and remedial massage (which is a passive form of exercise) do have calming and straightening-out effects. If you decide to take up any of these techniques while having McTimoney chiropractic treatment, it is important to discuss the matter with your chiropractor first so that you don't inadvertently undo the good the treatment is doing you.

The Side-effects of Drugs

One final subject comes under self-help. You may not associate your aches and pains with the prescription drugs you may be taking for a condition which seems totally unrelated to the reason for your visit to a chiropractor. Yet every drug known has an adverse side-effect on someone. While it may affect only one person in 10,000, you may be that one. Tell your chiropractor what you are taking, even if it's an apparently 'safe' drug bought over the counter. While he or she will not interfere with your doctor's prescription, side-effects are published in easily available pharmaceutical lists. If necessary, you may well be able to ask your doctor or chemist for another drug that has a different formula but the same palliative effect, and to which you have no adverse reaction. Do not simply keep on with repeat prescriptions. New and better formulae are being continually researched. Better still, be positive; follow your chiropractor's lead and get to the cause of the problem.

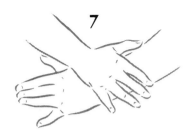

7

TREATING CHILDREN

The gentle McTimoney approach is particularly suitable
for children and even infants. In fact, McTimoney
chiropractors believe that treatment should ideally be
given soon after birth, to correct any misalignments at the
start and lay the foundations for the development of a
healthy spine and nervous system. Although the bones are
not properly formed at birth, stresses in the soft tissue,
perhaps from a difficult birth process, can develop into
spinal problems as the baby grows. (Mothers, of course,
can also benefit from treatment both during pregnancy and
after the physical strains and stresses of giving birth.)

The McTimoney view is that, after the birth check-up,
infants should be assessed about twice more before starting
to walk – since any existing pelvic misalignment can be
compounded when walking starts, and can cause the
spine, knee and other joints to compensate. (Many adult

musculo-skeletal problems have their origins in untreated childhood subluxations.) General health also benefits: an American study in 1989 compared the child patients of 200 paediatricians with 200 children under chiropractic care: the health of those who had seen chiropractors was notably superior to that of those brought up under standard medical care – with fewer ear infections, allergies and cases of tonsillitis, and less occasion to use medication.

A number of McTimoney chiropractors have a special interest in treating children, a fact borne out by the existence of a weekly paediatric clinic in Northampton run by the College, where students can observe the treatment of babies and children. (Open to the general public the rest of the week, this clinic is set within a large medical practice whose doctors refer both adult and child patients for McTimoney treatment when appropriate.)

Chiropractic can relieve a surprisingly wide range of childhood conditions, from colic to rheumatic diseases, and even behavioural difficulties and hyperactivity.

One paediatric chiropractor, Fiona Macrae, says:

Mothers report that the physiotherapist notices a difference in their babies, and that they're making good progress – but this could be because they are growing and developing anyway; there's no objective way of knowing. The way we feel about it is to have faith in the treatment and know that every time we treat, we are actually helping to restore the nervous system to as optimum function as we can.

As with any adult patient, a child visiting a McTimoney chiropractor will first be assessed. The practitioner will take a full history from the parents and will also question the child, if the child is old enough to answer. The chiropractor will tell the parents whether there is a spinal dysfunction which can be adjusted or, if appropriate, refer them to a physiotherapist or doctor. He or she will observe the child's co-ordination and personality. Sometimes it is necessary to reassure parents who feel guilty about children suffering from accidents or inherited problems.

Children, like adults, are given a whole-body assessment and treatment at each session. One satisfied mother (a hospital nurse) comments:

It's the subtlety of the treatment that makes it perfect for children – perfect for me, too, because I don't like cracking and crunching. And I've been impressed with the holistic approach. The chiropractor doesn't just treat symptoms as such; she checks the whole body every time, and makes adjustments where she needs to.

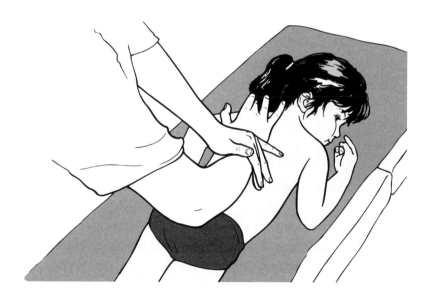

Most children thoroughly enjoy being treated and, since they have not yet acquired the fixed postural habits which can slow down adult recovery, they respond very rapidly. If appropriate, the chiropractor will also advise on posture, exercise, how to carry school bags, and so on.

What Can McTimoney Chiropractic Help?

Birth Trauma

The birth process itself can affect spinal alignment; indeed, subluxation can occasionally occur in the womb – for example when there is insufficient amniotic fluid, or in the case of multiple births. Even a normal delivery can affect the baby's spine, especially if there is an awkward presentation (for example if the baby emerges bottom first). Chiropractic is particularly recommended after difficult deliveries, especially those requiring the use of a vaunts (suction of the baby's head) or forceps, which can easily squash or twist the baby's vulnerable skull and neck.

Typical subluxations in babies occur in the pelvis, cervical spine (neck), lower thoracic spine, cranial (skull) and facial bones.

Parents need not be alarmed at the idea of manipulating a small baby's spine: spinal adjustments, carried out with the fingertips, are feather-light – and all the more effective for that, since they set up no reaction of pain and muscular tension. 'Babies love to receive chiropractic treatment,' comments Dawn Akers, an assistant at the paediatric clinic who also runs her own clinic. 'They will often break out into a huge smile, giggle and laugh, and apparently be experiencing peace and bliss. A crying baby will stop crying during treatment, and a fractious baby will settle down.'

■ **One of Dawn Akers' cases involved an induced delivery during which the forceps squashed the infant's right hand against his forehead, causing bruising to the left side of his face. At nine weeks, when his worried mother brought him to the clinic, his left eye was not closing properly, his head movements were restricted, and the muscles on the left side of his mouth were flaccid so that he could not suck properly. The hospital diagnosis was 'facial palsy'.**

Dawn Akers found misalignments to the right frontal and zygomatic bones of the face and in the cervical spine (the neck). After his first treatment, to his mother's great delight, there was an immediate improvement in his head and neck movements. His smile was more even, showing better nerve control in the facial muscles, and his eye had started closing better. Monthly treatments continued to produce a steady improvement. ■

Many difficulties might be avoided if it were standard practice for new babies to have an expert spinal check-up. After treating a woman through pregnancy, Fiona Macrae was asked to see her eight-week-old premature twins, one of whom was not feeding properly.

Whether [the baby] had difficulty swallowing, or whether it was her digestion I don't know – and she couldn't tell us! I gave her a whole-body assessment, just as for an adult but suitably modified, and treated where necessary. As a result her whole system began to function better, and there was a very definite improvement.

There are numbers of mothers who are very grateful to McTimoney chiropractors. Cases of birth damage successfully treated include 'floppy baby' syndrome and Erb's palsy – a flaccid arm due to nerve damage, possibly caused by the use of suction during birth.

■ One little girl, treated from two months old, was completely recovered by 10 months; and another, treated between the ages of 6 and 10 months old, was saved the trauma of an amputation. Another remarkable case is that of a boy of 15 whose bone growth was delayed by two years. He came to the chiropractor with a fractured right hand; on assessment, the chiropractor learned that he had been delivered face up, and deduced that the resulting misalignments of his skull and facial bones could be affecting his pituitary gland. After six treatments he had grown two and a half inches, and his face had noticeably changed shape for the better. ■

■ Little Zoe had a troubled start with a urinary tract infection at three weeks old; four weeks later her mother Peni discovered a lump on her spine. The baby was also having bouts of projectile vomiting and screaming fits. Peni was recommended to see Madeleine Brzeski, head of the paediatric clinic in Northampton. 'It was extraordinary how quickly there was a big change in her,' says Peni. Madeleine found a curvature in Zoe's spine, and that the lump was caused by a gross misalignment in the lower spine; she recommended taking Zoe to a consultant for a further opinion. By the time they saw the consultant, after four to five months of weekly treatments, there was a slight lump (one vertebra was more pronounced) but no sign of a spinal problem.

Although the doctors considered that the spinal misalignment and urinary tract infection were unrelated, Madeleine felt the two problems were linked, though which had come first it was hard to say. Peni comments: 'At the first treatment I couldn't believe how gentle it was. I was used to seeing hospital staff pulling her legs apart, and the difference was gigantic. I just knew my child was in safe and loving hands.' ■

Asthma, Bronchial Disorders and Allergy

Children with respiratory disorders including asthma usually respond well to chiropractic; it is obviously preferable to free the nervous system to function fully, rather than loading the body with drugs.

■ Typical is the case of a 15-month-old girl with persistent night coughing; she was diagnosed as asthmatic and prescribed Ventolin, though she never used this. After three chiropractic treatments she had no more asthmatic coughing; this improvement had been maintained when she had a check-up at the age of five. ■

Asthma often accompanies other allergies:

■ The patient of a McTimoney chiropractor mentioned that her little boy suffered from asthma and eczema, and the chiropractor offered to take a look at him. It had not occurred to the mother that chiropractic treatment could help, but as he had had a few tumbles recently she thought it would do no harm.

When he came to the clinic, 11-year-old Peter was using an inhaler once a day and was suffering from eczema and urticaria (skin irritation), both of which he had had from an early age. He was otherwise reasonably healthy. In assessing him, the chiropractor found that the T1 (the first thoracic vertebra at the top of the back, which is often involved in cases of asthma) was noticeably out of alignment, and adjusted this as part of his whole-body treatment.

When Peter returned the following week he announced that he had only used the inhaler twice in the interval, and his mother reported that he had been a lot calmer. At his next treatment a fortnight later he had continued to improve: he was hardly using his inhaler at all, and his eczema was clearing up. Peter had three treatments in all, and was advised to return for top-up treatments at intervals to maintain the improvement. ■

Bed-wetting and Bladder Problems

Bed-wetting is often associated with emotional problems (and can, of course, cause them) but it may well stem from purely physical problems in the lumbar spine, where the nerve supply to the bladder leaves the spinal cord. Children suffering from low back pain following a fall often wet their beds. Madeleine Brzeski has treated several such children for back pain, and cessation of bed-wetting has been a welcome side-effect. She has only seen one child specifically for bed-wetting, 'a six year-old who was becoming very embarrassed because she wanted to stay with friends. She had a pelvic problem, and after two treatments she was fine.'

Other urinary problems may also respond to chiropractic, such as the frequent need to pass water, especially where no medical cause can be found.

Colic and Bowel Problems

Disorders of the gut quite often relate to a vertebral problem. In 1984 the Danish Chiropractors Association carried out a questionnaire study on the infant patients of chiropractors, with the aim of finding out for which ailments infants under 12 months were taken to chiropractors. Of the 189 (of 270) parents who responded, 132 had brought their babies, averaging six weeks old, with infant colic. Of these, 72 (54 per cent) were cured, and 48 (37 per cent) improved; 12 (9 per cent) showed no change, and none was worse. The change in symptoms occurred after an average of two to three treatments, showing that this was not a case of the problem simply 'burning out'. Even if the 30 per cent of parents who did not reply were not helped, this is still a high rate of improvement.

■ **Madeleine Brzeski successfully treated a case after the mother had tried all the dietary possibilities. When she examined the baby, she found a problem in the neck – the neck is almost always involved in colic. 'When I adjusted it, it felt as if a ripple went through the baby's body as it relaxed; the baby was obviously holding a lot of tension there – it had had quite a difficult birth.'** ■

Chiropractic can be equally successful with constipation in certain cases:

■ One 10-month-old girl had, since birth, had bowel movements only every four to six days, accompanied by pain. Following chiropractic treatment she began regular daily motions, and had no further problems. ■

Cerebral Palsy and Neurological Problems

Madeleine Brzeski's work with cerebral palsy cases can be called pioneering. The families of these children express enormous enthusiasm for the effects of treatment. Unfortunately, ongoing weekly treatment is best, so there is a big demand for the free weekly clinic provided by the McTimoney College. A trust fund has been set up with the aim of founding more paediatric clinics on the same lines.

Dr David Buckler, a doctor specializing in Sports Medicine (who also lectures on research at the College) says: 'With cerebral palsy the effects are similar to those of physiotherapy in that it prevents contractures, shortening of muscles, it keeps the muscle balance and helps keep them mobile.' McTimoney chiropractors believe they are doing more than this by also stimulating, restoring and maintaining optimum nerve function. In other words, it is a treatment for the nervous system. With brain damage, therefore, while treatment will not provide a cure, it can help children to reach their personal potential and prevent further damage from poor posture, poor balance and muscle spasms. Other neurological conditions that can benefit include dyslexia, dyspraxia, Down's syndrome and autism. Children with spina bifida can be treated where there is no protrusion of the spinal cord.

Madeleine Brzeski points out, 'When normal children are brain-damaged through an accident, other parts of the brain will take over, up to the age of seven (sometimes 12). The nervous system has an amazing way of almost regenerating.' If children receive treatment soon after birth, the still immature nervous system is stimulated to create better connections between the brain and the body. Fiona Macrae treated one of Madeleine Brzeski's patients in her absence, a child of four who had been treated regularly for two years; she remarked that to the untrained eye no one would know she had cerebral palsy. As Dr Buckler says, more research is needed, and this would seem to be a very suitable subject.

■ **Madeleine Brzeski began working with disabled children by chance, when a mother asked her to see her 18-month-old boy. He had been unresponsive to stimuli since birth, and could not sit, stand, crawl, make eye contact or vocalize. An MRI scan showed that his brain was not developing normally, and at one year old a paediatrician told his parents he was unlikely ever to walk or communicate. He was allocated various forms of specialist help, but when Madeleine first saw him he had developed scoliosis, and had no muscle tone or limb control.**

Madeleine herself was 'staggered' at the effects of her McTimoney treatment. After eight weekly treatments he was sitting with support, holding his head up well and focusing his eyes better; his leg and abdominal muscles were developing. After 10 treatments he was standing with support and 'chatting'. As treatments continued he developed more and more co-ordination and muscle control; a year later he was free of medication, active, vocal and standing. He could participate in family activities with both sounds and actions, and respond to simple commands – not a perfect child, but a responsive and much happier one. ■

■ Mrs Bell, grandmother of a two-year old with cerebral palsy, noticed remarkable changes in little Megan after 10 weekly treatments at the paediatric clinic. At her hospital Child Development Group she saw the effects of McTimoney treatment on two other toddlers, and decided to try it. Megan was also seeing a physiotherapist and being taken through her physiotherapy exercises daily at home. The physiotherapist was dubious about McTimoney treatment at first – but Mrs Bell's doctor, having himself been treated by Madeleine Brzeski, was all for it. The effects on Megan, according to Mrs Bell, were 'brilliant'.

I was a bit sceptical at first, but it does work. Her movements were very limited, but she is now beginning to move her legs better and kick herself round in a circle. And she's trying to crawl. She loves the treatment, and has a good hour and a half sleep after each time. ■

■ A two-and-a-half-year-old boy was brought to Dawn Akers, suffering from brain and nerve damage. At six months he had been unable to lift his head well due to poor neck muscle tone, and his condition was diagnosed as 'progressive spinal atrophy'. At nine months, an accident at the hospital left him with damage to the temporal and occipital lobes of the brain, producing generalized muscular atrophy and loss of motor function. At his first visit, although he was already having physiotherapy he was suffering from scoliosis (curvature of the spine) due to lying for long hours in a cot on a ventilator.

Dawn found that the scoliosis was caused by a tilted pelvis; after two months' weekly treatment, realigning the pelvis had greatly reduced the scoliosis and the little boy was able briefly to hold his head up without support. His hip joints were more flexible and his spinal muscle tone had slightly increased.

This was not going to be a total cure: Dawn's aim was to realign the pelvis and spine so that when he came to use a walking frame his body would be in the best possible position. Since receiving chiropractic treatment his parents feel more confident, knowing that his body maintains a good alignment and that his nervous system can work as well as possible. ■

Sometimes other neurological problems can be helped quite dramatically:

■ One unhappy 13-year-old was brought to see Madeleine Brzeski with the dire label 'non-specific neurological deficiency syndrome'. She had a reading age of four, was overweight, aggressive and violent, and lacked sufficient co-ordination even to dress herself. After a few treatments, Madeleine put her on a sugar- and additive-free diet; her immediate weight loss made her look and feel much better. Madeleine did a lot of cranial work on her, manipulating the bones of the face and skull, as well as working on her very curved spine. Her behaviour began to settle down; she became relaxed and started sleeping well. After about nine months of treatment her reading had improved to the level of a 10-year-old; she could dance, skip – and use a computer. And she could look forward to being an integrated member of society. ■

Glue Ear and Hearing Problems

Glue ear is a common problem which if left untreated can last years and cause much misery, but it can respond speedily to chiropractic. Like so many childhood problems, it is chiefly associated with subluxations in the neck (at the atlas and axis), apparently caused during birth. The younger the child, the quicker the problem can clear up. Carried out early enough, a single treatment may be enough to stimulate the body to work normally.

Other hearing defects can of course stem from a variety of causes, but where there is a definite vertebral problem cures and improvements – though rare – have been known to occur (as in D D Palmer's famous first cure). The connection may not always be obvious, however: John McTimoney treated a 12-year-old girl who had become deaf following mumps at the age of two; after six weekly treatments she was able to throw away the hearing aid she had worn for three years.

Headaches, Migraines and Sinus Problems

Chronic headaches or migraines can have a variety of causes, including food sensitivities and eyesight problems. They may also result from subluxations in the atlas and axis bones at the top of the spine; these can result from stress – sometimes emotional but often physical, such as carrying heavy school bags. Sometimes the cause goes back to birth:

■ **An eight-year-old boy had been experiencing severe headaches and right-sided neck pain. On history-taking, the chiropractor learned that he had had a difficult birth during** which the umbilical cord had become wrapped around his neck; he'd been pushed backwards up the birth canal where the cord untwisted, and then 're-birthed'. The chiropractor found that his atlas was rotated; after three treatments the boy had no headaches and felt much better all round. In addition his vision had improved, he was concentrating better at school and his teachers noticed that his attention span had increased. ■

If a happy child below the age of speech suddenly becomes fractious and difficult, this may be his only way of telling you that he or she has a pain or headache. A spinal examination may be well worthwhile, particularly if the child has had a fall before the change in behaviour. Falls can also lead to altered behaviour and uncharacteristic aggressiveness in older children, especially if the neck has been affected.

■ A seven-year-old girl was brought to a chiropractor suffering from stomach-aches and frontal headaches on waking most weekdays, together with pins and needles in her hands. She had suffered these symptoms for about a year. Her mother had recently remarried and had a new baby, and thought the cause was emotional. On the point of taking the child to a psychiatrist, she decided to see a McTimoney chiropractor first. Chiropractic history-taking revealed that at the age of 18 months the child had fallen, hitting her head.

Examination showed subluxations of all the neck vertebrae, and the left jaw-joint was misaligned, as was the right lachrymal bone at the inner corner of the eye. The girl had four treatments, and at the final consultation had experienced only two headaches and one episode of stomach-ache in the previous two months. Also, the realization that the problem was physical, not emotional, was a great relief to the mother. ■

Sinus problems often result from misalignment in the facial bones, and treatment for this can also be very effective.

Hyperactivity and Behavioural Disorders

Two pilot studies conducted in Texas in 1974 and 1975 confirmed that spinal adjustments can help children with emotional, behavioural and neurological problems; the problems helped included asthma, anxiety, low mental stamina, inability to concentrate, hyperactivity and discipline problems.[1]

Hyperactivity is often associated with sensitivity to food (particularly sugar) and additives. Many hyperactive children have had a stressful birth, and when examined by chiropractors are often found to have an abnormally large number of spinal problems, particularly in the neck and lower back. Whether these cause the hyperactivity or are caused by it is not known, but treating them often helps to calm children down. As with asthma, the biomechanical factor may be one element in the whole syndrome, and when that element is dealt with the child stands a much better chance of coping.

■ **One desperate mother took her eight-year-old daughter to a chiropractor, suffering from lack of co-ordination, reading difficulties, hyperactivity and bed-wetting; in seven treatments she improved considerably. Interestingly, the mother was not convinced that her improvement related to the child's spine. Then, after a fall, her daughter's behaviour regressed, but once again settled after chiropractic treatment. This time the mother had to acknowledge that chiropractic was responsible. ■**

Growing children are notoriously susceptible to falls and bumps which are usually regarded as a normal part of growing up. But developing bones and joints are vulnerable, and no chiropractor would regard a mother as over-anxious if she took her child for a check-up after a bad tumble. A heavy impact on a hard surface can throw the spine and other joints out of alignment which, untreated, can lead to trouble later on. In fact, the sooner treatment is sought, the quicker the healing and the longer-lasting the results will be.

Chiropractors, like osteopaths and physiotherapists, can find themselves dealing with the results of school sport and games injuries, such as ankle problems and peripheral joint strains. Many would like the opportunity to do more preventative work, such as simply checking that there are no congenital problems such as hyper-mobile joints, which often go undiagnosed and cause children (and adults) major problems when engaging in physical activities.

Some parents can be over-ambitious for their children's physical prowess, and while the musculo-skeletal system is still developing there is a risk of causing long-term damage through over-exertion. In fact any backaches or joint pains in a child should never be dismissed as 'growing pains'; there is always a reason for pain.

Some chiropractors have developed their interest in the profession as a result of childhood experience. Tony Gilmore, for example, first met John McTimoney at the age of nine, when he was taken to him for a knee problem the doctors had failed to resolve.

*I remember thinking during the treatment that not much
could have happened since I didn't feel anything, and
I rather thought my folks were being taken for a ride.
However when I woke up next morning ... I realized
something had occurred. When the knee problem cleared
up after only two treatments I accepted it as normal.
Afterwards I used to visit Mac for bi-annual maintenance
treatments.*

■ **Dawn Akers treated a typical knee problem in a nine-year-old; he also had pain in the right groin, and Dawn found that
the cause was a tilted pelvis; the knee joints had become
misaligned as a result of compensation. He was completely
better after three treatments.** ■

Knee problems often accompany a pelvic misalignment,
and chiropractic seems to work very well both in relieving
symptoms and dealing with their cause. Very active
children may need maintenance treatment every few
months.

The connection between the knees and the pelvis is not
always obvious, not only to parents but also to the
medical profession:

■ **Little Lucy was about 18 months old when a health visitor
noticed that her feet turned inwards; she was referred to an
orthopaedic hospital where it was also noticed that she was
knock-kneed. She saw a physiotherapist once a month and
was given daily exercises which made little difference, while
plastic heel cups in her shoes hurt her feet and caused
blisters. By the age of four, her feet were so painful she found
it difficult to ride a bike or walk far, and running caused her
to fall over her feet. Medical advice was that she would get**

better eventually; if not, surgery could be considered which would involve breaking and re-setting the bones from knee to ankle and hip to knee – a painful operation with a poor prognosis, apart from requiring weeks in plaster and months of physiotherapy. Her parents could not contemplate this.

Lucy's grandmother suggested that McTimoney chiropractic might help, and they decided to give it a try. In September 1995, when Lucy was six and a half, they took her to see Stan Harding. He observed that her spine was not straight, due to a tilted and rotated pelvis which caused her body balance to be uneven, pushing the legs out of line. She improved after her first treatment and continued to improve with each session. By December 1995, Lucy was walking and running normally, and in 1998 her mother confirms that she has maintained the improvement: she can happily skate, cycle, run, skip and take long walks. Her mother says:

Lucy finds the McTimoney treatment comfortable; sometimes early on she would have side-effects – she could be emotional, tired or giggly for a day or so after. Now she likes to go for treatment, and if she falls on her back or her leg aches, she asks to go. Her feet are a much better shape, her ankles do not lean over so much, her spine is noticeably straighter. She has much more physical confidence and likes participating in sports. I didn't want her legs to be broken, so I believe if she hadn't had McTimoney chiropractic her legs would be just as bad now, if not worse. ■

Young people often suffer from aches and pains which are not helped by medical treatment:

■ A lad of 14 had severe, constant lower backache, as well as headaches. An orthopaedic consultant diagnosed Scheuermann's kyphosis; all he could do was to advise the boy to give up sports – which was devastating, as he 'lived' for sport. He had nine McTimoney treatments over five months for a pelvic tilt and rotation; these reduced his backache to only a feeling of weakness in the lumbar area. During the next two months he resumed participating in sports, though aware of his limits and the need to return for preventative treatments when necessary. ■

McTimoney chiropractors also find themselves treating the after-effects of accidents:

■ A boy of 12 suffered from a torn Achilles tendon, probably caused during rugby, which had not healed after three months; the doctor told him to rest. The chiropractor found that he also had a pelvic and thoracic rotation; after three weekly whole-body treatments, all his symptoms had cleared up. ■

■ A 10-year-old girl had a TMJ (temporomandibular joint) problem after being in a traffic accident. Her jaw moved to the right on opening and she had developed a lisp which made her self-conscious and withdrawn. With bi-monthly treatment her jaw movement improved, the lisping went, and she interacted better with her friends. ■

Rheumatic Disorders: Still's Disease

Arthritic and rheumatic problems in children can be painful and disabling, and chiropractic treatment should only be sought with the co-operation of the doctor in charge of the case.

Madeleine Brzeski recounted what seems like a remarkable instance of medical open-mindedness (though the consultant concerned, motivated by what was best for his patient, did not consider it particularly remarkable):

■ When 13-year-old Stephen fell ill with Still's Disease (a form of inflammatory arthritis in children) his mother, hearing that Madeleine had had some success with rheumatoid arthritis in adults, spoke to the consultant paediatrician, who invited Madeleine in for a talk about her work.

Medical management of Still's Disease includes the use of anti-inflammatory drugs during the acute phase and ensuring that the child's joints become as little deformed as possible by protecting the limbs with splints and plaster casts. Finally, once the acute pain and discomfort have died down, mobility has to be restored to the joints and strength to the wasted muscles. It was in this last area that the consultant felt that Madeleine could help, particularly as what she was offering seemed preferable to the boy's other options – either three short sessions of physiotherapy a week, or removal to a specialist hospital some distance away.

Madeleine started working with Stephen while he was going through the inflammatory stage of the disease. He was given conventional medication and was in plaster for a short time, but the hospital allowed Madeleine to help reduce the inflammation with cold compresses rather than using their own hot wax treatment. They also co-operated with her suggestion of putting him on a diet free of sugar, additives and red meat, and the physiotherapist taught Madeleine the remedial exercises he himself would normally have carried out.

Instead of going to a special hospital Stephen was sent home under Madeleine's care. She treated him for just over a year, daily at first. Madeleine stresses:

With a disease like this, we don't work specifically on any one area. It is now recognized that the nervous system communicates directly with the immune system, and so we are stimulating the body to heal itself.

By the end of the year Stephen's blood tests were clear and he returned to school. He started playing rugby again, against Madeleine's better judgement, and the disease returned. Madeleine treated him again, in conjunction with the local doctor and the hospital; all three kept in communication, and Stephen recovered once more. ■

Still's Disease normally burns itself out by adulthood, but usually by then some joint deformity has set in. By the age of 19 Stephen had no joint deformity whatsoever, and passed a medical to join the army. It is impossible to say for certain whether he did better with chiropractic care than he would otherwise have done. The consultant commented that Stephen, who had had relatively severe acute Still's Disease, recovered remarkably well. 'One can't say whether chiropractic was better than conventional physiotherapy or not, because it's not been tested out in any numbers,' he says, 'but simple common sense would suggest that the amount of time Madeleine was able to offer would be better than anything I could organize.'

This is one of many areas in which properly conducted research might be of real benefit. Since then, Madeleine Brzeski has treated several more such cases, with equally good results.

Scoliosis, Backache and Postural Problems

Slight scoliosis (an S-shaped curve in the spine) can easily occur in growing children, appearing after the age of 10 as a result of poor posture (particularly standing with the weight on one leg) or the strain of activities like ballet, sports, gym and carrying heavy school bags. It is most commonly found in girls around the age of puberty, and the sooner it is treated the better. Although some people have scoliosis with no pain or difficulties, the condition may develop into a serious deformity.

Very severe cases may need hospital treatment such as plaster corsets or surgery, but a chiropractor will be able to tell if the spine can be treated chiropractically. Often the problem is pelvic in origin rather than spinal; once the subluxated pelvis is adjusted, the lumbar and thoracic curves begin to realign themselves, and more invasive treatment may be avoided.

Children can easily develop postural problems, not necessarily through their own fault. School desks, chairs and computer centres are often ill-designed, and in 1997 the National Back Pain Association conducted a worrying survey which found that an increasing number of children are developing back problems relating to carrying heavy school bags and sports gear. Up to 80 per cent of schoolchildren were found to be carrying badly designed bags, or carrying them incorrectly. Eleven- to 12-year-olds were carrying an average of 12–13 per cent of their body weight, and in some cases up to 25 kg – over 60 per cent of their body weight. They were also, either from following fashion or because of the design of the bags, tending to carry them over one shoulder instead of having the weight evenly distributed.

All of these factors can lead to back problems, shoulder pain and headaches. They take a heavy toll on the spine, potentially leading to early disc degeneration. Today, orthopaedic consultants are seeing an increasing number of children with back problems. An occasional McTimoney assessment and treatment will straighten out the spine and give the child a sense of what good posture actually feels like – and that it feels better than slouching or slumping!

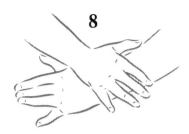

8

TREATING ANIMALS

As with all the aspects of the McTimoney story, animal manipulation has come a very long way since John McTimoney's first successes in the 1960s. At the time of writing (late 1998) there are over 20 McTimoney animal practitioners working in co-operation with vets with a variety of patients, from race-horses and show dogs to domestic pets and farm animals. The attitude of the veterinary profession has changed radically: they are aware that animals, like humans, can develop spinal and other problems for which manipulation is appropriate, and for which there is no conventional solution. An increasing number are happy to refer their clients to practitioners whom they know to be suitably skilled and qualified. Some osteopaths, BCA chiropractors and physiotherapists also treat animals, and the Oxford College of Chiropractic (the McTimoney-Corley group) also offers a training in animal manipulation. However, the McTimoney College is currently unique in offering an externally validated post-graduate Diploma in animal manipulation. This course was designed in co-operation with the Royal College of Veterinary Surgeons, includes vets among its lecturers and is open to vets (among other suitably qualified candidates – *see Chapter 3, page 53*).

Under British law it is still illegal for a non-veterinary manipulator to treat an animal without the approval of a veterinary surgeon, but this approval is much easier to obtain than it once was. If approached direct, McTimoney practitioners check that the client has their vet's permission, and asks them to obtain it if necessary. In the case of a new patient it is natural that the vet may want to see the animal first to rule out other veterinary problems, or perhaps to get X-rays or an orthopaedic opinion. However, once the vet knows both the animal and the practitioner, a telephone call to the vet may be enough before seeing the chiropractor.

Tony Gilmore, a highly experienced animal chiropractor, finds that:

Vets are much more ready now to accept outsiders doing procedures they don't understand. A number of vets today are practising complementary therapies themselves, including homoeopathy and acupuncture. There's a generalized change in scientific philosophy – for example the discovery of quantum theory and the uncertainty principle in science, which are comparatively recent concepts, have paved the way for an acceptance of the science-art combination of complementary therapies. Chiropractic is a combination of art and science and manual dexterity. There's an easy way and a hard way, a way that works with

The Essentials of McTimoney Chiropractic

the body and a way that works against it. It's much more comfortable to do it the easy way.

The 'easy way' consists of adjustments, based on the toggle-torque-recoil technique, which work in co-operation with the animal's spine and muscles, causing minimal discomfort. Just as with humans, treatment will include a whole-body assessment: the spine, pelvis and joints are analysed for any misalignments or muscle spasm.

Treating an animal, says Dana Green (who treats both humans and animals), 'is no different from treating a person, except that the animal's spine is aligned horizontally instead of vertically, so you can't really get to the front of the pelvis'. Some animals apparently make better patients than people and they recover quickly. As Dana Green points out, animals often have a healthier lifestyle than their owners:

They have a very strong instinctive desire to be well, and they know you're coming to make them well, even the first time. In nature, a dog who doesn't have four good legs will starve, a horse in the wild that can't keep up with the herd is picked off by predators. They don't get sick pay or sympathy, so they have a far stronger intuitive leaning to get better. Sometimes they'll indicate the spot that needs adjusting. A horse will actually push its back towards me as if to say 'this is the bit, here.' Most of them become exceptionally calm, almost dreamy, and they respond speedily.

One chiropractor describes horses 'going into trance' at a colleague's touch. Tony Gilmore feels there may be more than one reason for this. 'One is that any procedure that's done on a horse produces an endorphin response. And I think some people have got a good rapport with horses and others haven't.' Equine chiropractor Mark Windsor says:

For every 50–60 horses that I deal with I probably get one which objects. The vast majority almost innately know you are helping them; when you start working even on a very nervous horse it has quite a soporific effect and they start to relax and drop the head, and you very often hear them breathe out as they relax. There's not many that don't enjoy it.

Animals who already know their chiropractors certainly make it clear that they are pleased to see them. One chiropractor describes a dog she had seen once 'dragging his owner into my yard' on the second visit. Ian Miller treats a number of dogs, but has never been bitten – 'A dog once pressed a tooth on one of my fingers during a treatment, but it was to let me know he felt sore.'

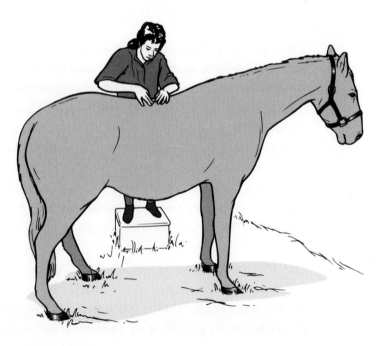

Occasionally chiropractors come across stroppy patients (goats seem particularly prone to stroppiness), but if they do get kicked it's usually a sign that something is seriously wrong.

When to Treat Animals

Owners who care about their animals soon notice when something is amiss. It can be as obvious as limping, or a dog crying in pain, but there may be more subtle changes in the animal's gait or behaviour. Limb-dragging, lop-sidedness, reduced performance or uneven wear of shoes in horses are common indications that something has gone awry. So are changes in temperament: uncharacteristic bad temper or moodiness for which no other cause can be found, unexpected resistances in horses such as napping, rearing and refusing – all these are ways in which animals express discomfort.

Animals with a particular weak spot may need regular maintenance treatment. It is also recommended for animals, like humans, to have a check-up after a difficult labour and after any kind of surgery requiring a general anaesthetic. When a limp body is handled under anaesthesia it is easy for twists and subluxations to occur. For example, chiropractor Margie Craib treated a fairly elderly fox terrier; following castration (necessitated by a small penile growth) he refused to go for walks, or even to cock his leg. When he came back for his second treatment, he was already fully recovered.

Horses probably form the largest part of most McTimoney animal practices; horse owners, particularly those who compete, are extremely aware of the need to keep their animals on top form, and notice at once when they are under par. The same goes for show dogs and racing dogs. McTimoney chiropractors find themselves doing a good deal of work on such animals which, though not in pain, are not performing at their best. They also do 'preventative maintenance or fine-tuning' before important races or events.

Domestic pets and farm animals can benefit, too. 'There's enormous potential among domestic animals, if more vets knew more about it,' says Ian Miller. 'The clients seem happy and the animals are very happy with the service!' Dogs, cows, sheep, goats, pigs, ferrets, even hamsters and the occasional duck – any vertebrate animal can suffer from subluxations, often through a fall, some kind of strain or an accident. Cats, with their enviable litheness, are perhaps the least common patients; the occasional aged, arthritic cat has been helped to regain mobility, but chiropractors are most likely to see cats after road accidents, when treatment can help in their recovery.

It is rare for zoo animals to be treated, since they are not used to being handled and have to be sedated. This makes treatment much more difficult since the body does not respond to adjustment in the same way as it does when conscious. (Occasionally horses are sedated before treatment, but McTimoney chiropractors prefer them to be alert and reactive.)

As some of the following stories show, many animals who could not be helped by conventional veterinary treatment have been spared an untimely death by the gentle hands of a McTimoney practitioner.

What Can McTimoney Chiropractic Help?

Dogs

Dogs' lives have their risks. Working dogs and performance dogs in particular have extra strains put on their physical systems. Lynda Clark, who has a large animal practice, mainly treats horses but gets a fair number of dog patients, too, including police dogs:

■ *Police dogs work quite hard, and have to jump huge heights in their training. I had one whose gait was most peculiar; his handler was worried he would have to retire him early, but he was fine after treatment. No significant abnormality showed up on his X-rays, although there was said to be some 'wear and tear'. In my terms, the pelvis was not correctly aligned and this, chiropractically, could account for the wear and tear and his peculiar gait.* ■

Lynda kept another police dog going who was threatened with early retirement due to his weak, uncoordinated gait:

■ *The vet suspected CDRM, a condition German Shepherds and other breeds get, where the nerve impulses are not getting through to the back legs very well. He was a very good worker and the police force were quite happy for him to have regular treatment, which kept him in active work for two years until his retirement – his handler was retiring at the same time.* ■

Racing greyhounds are subject to particular hazards. Constantly running round tracks in one direction is just one of the stresses on their musculo skeletal systems; they can also bump into each other while racing, causing quite serious knocks. Lynda Clark regularly treats the animals at a large greyhound kennel:

■ *One dog who normally holds the bends very well had had a knock in a race; he had started to run very wide and almost came to a stop while racing; the vet found nothing obviously wrong – but I found problems with his atlas and pelvis. After a couple of treatments he was back to form, and back to his normal 'tight' racing.*

Another greyhound had a bad tumble in a race, and was in a lot of pain with what appeared to be his neck – he was holding his head down and crying. The course vet found no broken bones, and gave him a painkiller. Two days later when I saw him he was still crying in pain, and had a very definite atlas rotation; after treatment he was rapidly more comfortable and went back to racing happily and successfully. ■

Sheepdogs are also subject to risks of various kinds both while training and working:

■ **One of Margie Craib's canine patients, a young sheepdog called Bess, had caught her hind leg in some wire when jumping over a fence.**

She was a very timid little dog, who had possibly been harshly treated during training, and she wouldn't leave her current owner's side. She had a twisted pelvis and problems in her lumbar region, which were put right in three sessions. She was very sweet; she gave me a lick at the end to say thank you very much. Dogs tend to be very expressive in their post-treatment behaviour!

Since then Bess has been very well, with an annual 'MOT' and a post-birth check-up after producing a litter; she has also become more outgoing. ■

Domestic dogs, too, are liable to falls and bumps, traffic accidents and disc degeneration:

■ A regular patient of Ian Miller's is Gemma, a Border Collie whose younger and bouncier Collie companion knocks her over at frequent intervals – though her problems may have started in the days when she was a working sheep-dog, a career which holds the risks of being knocked about by the sheep. Gemma clearly loves her treatment, standing still while Ian checks and adjusts her pelvis and the whole spine including the neck and back. After a final massage, she lies down in a state of relaxed bliss. ■

■ Neil Coode, a vet who refers a number of dogs to Ian, is happy with the results – from the time when Ian speedily and effectively treated Neil's own back after he had been dealing with a stroppy horse. His veterinary practice was already using a chiropractor for horses, and was looking for someone interested in treating dogs when Ian got in touch with him. He says:

Problems associated with the spine are very common among dogs, and there is not a lot you can do conventionally, apart from painkillers and anti-inflammatories, which don't really get to the root of the problem. Nowadays anything I think might involve the spine I would refer to Ian automatically. I have to see the animal first, in case something else is wrong – though occasionally if owners ring me up I'll send them straight to Ian. When dogs have chronic problems their owners will just tell me they're going for a chiropractic treatment.

Chiropractic can also alleviate some arthritic conditions. A dog may walk awkwardly because of arthritis, or adopt particular postures to alleviate the pain; these can become habitual and lead to muscle spasm in places quite remote from the arthritis itself. This situation can be treated chiropractically.

As they get older a lot of dogs get weakness in the spine and back legs and chiropractic can help them too. They don't all improve, but a proportion will improve or stop degenerating. At a rough estimate, I would say 70–80 per cent of the patients we send over have a good to very good result. Sometimes the results can be spectacular. I have had some cases that literally couldn't walk and have come out of treatment walking.

This was the case with Willie, a 'Battersea Bitsa' treated by Dana Green when he was six. Willie had been hit by a car early in his life, and his owner had noted that he had a twisted back though this apparently caused no problems. Then, one day when out hacking behind his owner on her horse, Willie completely collapsed; he was unable to walk and was clearly in great pain. Rest and painkillers had no effect; his distressed owners had almost decided to have him put out of his misery when they sought chiropractic treatment as a last resort. Dana found a considerable distortion in the pelvis, with a resultant misalignment in the lower lumbar vertebrae. Within 20 minutes of treatment Willie was able to get up and run about, to his owners' great joy. He made a complete recovery and lived another 10 years, enjoying his rabbiting in the countryside. ■

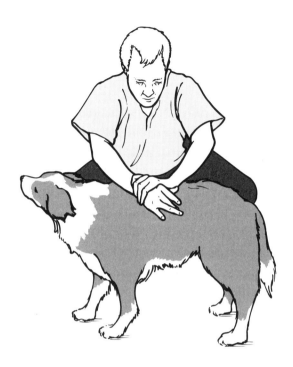

Farm Animals

McTimoney practitioners are trained to treat farm animals
– cattle, pigs, sheep and goats. 'Farmers are sometimes
sympathetic to their poor old cows,' comments Margie
Craib, 'particularly those who have back problems
themselves. Cows are not quite as biddable as horses, but I
do quite a bit of work with them, usually the show-quality
cows.' Margie treated one pedigree cow that wouldn't stand
up in the correct position for showing; she had problems in
her lower thoracic and lumbar region, which responded to
treatment. 'I have done several cows after calving; they
tend to have very big calves these days which puts a
tremendous pressure on them and can create problems.'

Sheep and goats can also suffer from post-partum problems, while rams and bulls have been treated for back problems occurring while covering females; it's not uncommon for them to slip, which can cause quite a jolt on a concrete yard.

■ A sheep called Nipper had started life as a pet lamb; he was part of a farming family and lived with the horses and chickens in a small paddock. When newly born he had been attacked by a fox, and had always had an odd kink along his back. One day, when he was around three, he collapsed, unable to stand or even to move. Veterinary treatment was sought, but after four days of antibiotics and steroids there was no improvement and his future was in serious doubt. However, his owners were recommended to try McTimoney manipulation: the first treatment included realigning his pelvis, which helped partially to straighten the twist in his back. He was then able to stand a little. After his second treatment a few days later he was running about in the paddock again. ■

■ Another animal which was nearly written off was a goat with a shoulder problem, who had been destined for the knacker's yard; when Margie Craib saw her she found that she had a treatable problem in the upper thoracic region. She was a particularly responsive patient – 'After each adjustment she turned her head round towards me and said "Me-eh!"' ■

■ Lynda Clark met one of her more unusual patients when she visited a farm to treat a dog; she was also asked to have a look at an unfortunate duck which had been lame on one leg for a couple of months (possibly after being attacked by a fox) and could only swim round in circles.

It was difficult to know where to start on a duck! But her owner held the 'sharp end', and I palpated her and felt how she would move, and where there was a block in her movement. I treated a problem low down on what seemed to be the pelvic girdle, and 24 hours later she was back to normal. ■

Horses

McTimoney chiropractors are now widely accepted in the horse world. Racing and eventing can put major stresses on an animal's system, and a number of McTimoney practitioners work closely with well-known race-horse trainers and owners – a practice which originated in the days when John McTimoney regularly treated horses belonging to the Royal Family. Shropshire-based Mark Windsor has been a full-time equine chiropractor for 15 years, and now regularly treats around 100 horses a week, from ordinary riding ponies to the horses of Olympic competitors including Michael Whitaker, Geoff Billington and Karen Dixon.

The rigours and stresses of training and competing can cause slight strains and subluxations which, although not always presenting in terms of major symptoms, can affect the horse's performance – at times quite dramatically.

'It is important to remember that many problems that occur in the horse's back are secondary to a problem somewhere else,' says Mark. For example, a horse may be incorrectly shod, or a low-grade lameness in a fetlock or a hock causes the horse to work out of balance, putting extra stress and strain on the structures in the back. As Mark explains:

A horse may come in with a lumbar problem, but this may be caused because he is shod too long in his toes, causing him to compensate in his action, stressing the back. It is no good only correcting the back without correcting the feet, because several weeks later the horse will be back with the same problem. The reverse is also true: a problem in the back will cause the horse to put more strain on the lower limbs and, again through compensation, damage other areas. A recent study in America shows that a lot of horses suffering forelimb tendon injury have primary problems in the back.

Whereas in the 1960s the general veterinary view was that a horse's spine was too solid to adjust, today a number of people in the horse world practise physiotherapy and other manipulative techniques as well as chiropractic. McTimoney's complete system involves adjusting most of the joints, including the pelvis, and a specific adjustment to the atlas, the first cervical bone just behind the head – a technique which can also calm a nervous animal.

■ **Lynda Clark treats horses and ponies of all kinds. One four-year-old New Forest pony had been rescued after her mother was killed in a road traffic accident. When the time came for her to be broken, she was found to be moving very oddly, particularly when a weight was put on her back – her legs wouldn't move in the right directions. As Lynda describes it, 'She was quite ataxic – the brain wasn't sending the right signals to the legs.' On examination, the number of problems she found made Lynda suspect that the pony had been involved in the accident that killed her mother:**

Although she had no obvious signs of injury at the time, she may have taken quite a tumble. She was wrong from the top of her neck and her head right down her back to the pelvis. She improved a lot after the first treatment; when I treated her again a couple of weeks later she was already much better. ■

How can the very light McTimoney technique affect something as strong as a horse's back? Mark Windsor comments:

In my experience, there is often a misunderstanding of what we are actually talking about. People use the expression 'putting your back out' or 'putting a vertebra out', but obviously that isn't what happens, it's anatomically impossible. What tends to happen is that when an animal gets a subluxation this produces subtle changes in function, in the soft tissue, rather than major movements of bone. When you are adjusting, you are not physically bludgeoning anything back into place; you are releasing a muscle spasm which allows the back to return to its normal integrity. The muscle responds to a light touch because you are applying an adjustment which sets up a series of reactions. The horse is actually self-adjusting. We are stimulating an area to respond, and you can see the muscle respond – there is a visible movement.

Horses also have their own ways of telling you they have backache. 'It's usually a change of temperament, like starting to refuse jumps,' says Lynda Clark. 'Or a very placid horse who suddenly won't have his head touched, or is miserable and bad-tempered.' Some animals will refuse to do things they normally have no problems with.

Equine vet Len Beech trains his own horses for endurance races. The star among them is Ben, a dark bay with thoroughbred blood, who was once a 'reject', destined for an early demise. Len took Ben to Lynda Clark.

■ **Lynda found that Ben had a lot of problems, particularly with the atlas and the lower back. How these originated is not known; as Lynda says,**

Problems can be due to bad handling, bad riding or trauma, but horses can do these things just around the field or being silly with each other! Temperamentally Ben was quite difficult, partly because of his background and partly because he was in discomfort and had been forced into doing things that were difficult and uncomfortable for him. Len Beech and his partner Pauline Dickie were very good at programming his rehabilitation.

Since Lynda began treating Ben regularly he has gone from strength to strength, and has become an endurance ride champion. 'He's now a very athletic horse, very supple,' says Len. 'Not so much wilful now as strong-willed, and at the age of 19 he's better than he ever has been.' ■

Clearly, Ben's progress has been due to a combination of the care of his owners and restoring his body to a peak state through the skill of McTimoney chiropractic at a crucial time in his life.

Several race-horse owners have longstanding working relationships with McTimoney chiropractors not just for remedial reasons, but in order to produce absolutely peak performance:

■ Probably one of the best race-horses Mark Windsor has treated over the past few years was the grey One Man. In 1995, while still a novice, One Man ran in the Sun Alliance Chase at Cheltenham, at the Cheltenham Festival. He hit the open ditch at the top of the hill, dragging his hind legs through it, and this no doubt wrenched his back quite badly. Running to the last fence, his stamina drained. If it had been a race of lesser importance the jockey would have pulled him up, but because he was favourite and still in third place he continued.

The next day the horse was a very sorry sight. He was extremely sore, and could hardly walk, standing with his hind legs right under him. It took fully three months of regular chiropractic treatment to get him sound again, but the following season he won the Hennessy Gold Cup, followed by two King George V Gold Cups, the second in a record time. His greatest triumph was the Queen Mother Champion Chase at Cheltenham in March 1998. He had regular chiropractic treatment to maintain his back because of the earlier injury, and to keep him performing to maximum performance. ■

Tony Gilmore also treats a number of first-class race-horses, sometimes checking them weekly for several weeks before a big race:

It's important to emphasize that just because owners have chiropractors in doesn't mean there's necessarily something wrong with that horse. You don't have to feel bad to feel better! You can be quite OK and yet be underfunctioning. Regular treatment can be a process of fine-tuning, like fine-tuning an engine. We are looking at optimum performance.

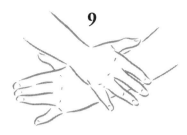

9

THE FUTURE OF McTIMONEY CHIROPRACTIC

Chiropractic is going through a metamorphosis, as chiropractic associations work towards agreed professional standards in all relevant fields. In the UK this accompanies implementation of the Chiropractor's Bill.

No one knows exactly what the future holds, but when discussing the possibilities and opportunities it seemed relevant to interview two key people: Ian Pearson, past principal of the McTimoney Chiropractic College, and Christina Cunliffe, new principal and chairman of the McTimoney Chiropractic Association. We begin with Ian Pearson.

Q: What do you see as the future of McTimoney chiropractic?

IP: I think we should begin our discussion with the situation here in the UK, and be much clearer about the immediate effects of the General Chiropractic Council (GCC) and registration. It is becoming increasingly difficult to keep the course to four years. The new honours degree course, if taken as a part-time course, may eventually spread over six years, plus an obligatory probationary year. This raises questions about continuity.

From a business point of view, I don't feel it is possible for the college to sustain a distance-learning mixed-mode course at that level on student income alone. These fees just will not cover delivery of the existing course as well as development of the new course – which is what we need to do. We have to find other sources of income. The Trust, which governs us under our charitable status, are looking at grants and awards of various types available in the charitable sector. But this, in the long-term, is unpredictable. We need other predictable, long-term funding that will give financial stability. So far none of these ideas has been brought to fruition, largely because there is neither the expertise within the College, nor the funds to bring in consultants.

I think the first priority would be the development of another college, a parallel course, using the work already done at Abingdon, thus spreading the cost of course development. My personal preference would be in the north – York or Harrogate. There are no chiropractic colleges north of Oxford, and yet we are consistently receiving students from well north of that. I am quite convinced there is a market to be exploited somewhere in Scotland, the Borders or North Wales.

Similarly I think the particular route that McTimoney chiropractic has taken will always have a limited market segment because at the moment the chiropractic world is dominated by the scientific/medical model. Those who are pursuing a different model will always have a minority share of the market.

McTimoney in Europe

My next move would therefore be to establish the UK McTimoney colleges as a European base, and look at either setting up a McTimoney college within mainland Europe, or bringing students from mainland Europe to a McTimoney college in the UK. It has not escaped my notice that at one point the Anglo-European College (AECC) had more than half its students coming in from Europe. There undoubtedly is a market in Europe for practitioners who are more inclined towards the intuitive end of the scale – that is the next market to look at – to develop the 'brand name' within mainland Europe.

However, there are concomitant issues, the primary one being the acceptability of the McTimoney training in European countries. It is very complicated in Europe because there are statutory requirements and professional requirements, and no common understanding between countries.

McTimoney in North America, Australia and the Far East

There is also the issue of the qualification being accepted in the United States, Canada and Australia. This has to be resolved before too much money is invested in developing a course which may not be acceptable outside certain specific areas. Acceptability and portability are important market forces.

It is already happening the other way round. We have been visited by Australia's Royal Melbourne Institute of Technology (RMIT), who are exporting chiropractic courses under franchise worldwide. We have had contact with their Principal on developing joint projects. At the moment there is an ex-AECC lecturer working in Melbourne who has offered to look at research projects for us. RMIT have already sold well into Japan and the Far East in particular, and are keen to establish a base in Europe. They do a lot by distance learning.

The Far East and China are worth exploring in the long-term. They are used to looking at things from a different medical perspective which is much more comparable with that found within the McTimoney framework. There are lots of other specialists whom we might be able to take on, but the market would be much tougher. None the less the potential is huge.

Franchising

I think it is important that we look at franchising the courses into areas such as the emerging countries and also to Eastern Europe, where I think there is a need and a commercial opportunity. We have already touched on this with visits to Bosnia and other places. The interest that we were getting was from doctors who wanted to re-train on a 'fast track'. At the time we could not offer them a fast-track course and they could not afford to come over here to do a part-time course. Now we are looking at a possible one- or two-year fast-track course – and I think there is a great gain to be made there.

Q: What about fast-track courses for British doctors?

IP: There seems to be a strong resistance within the profession to fast-track people. There is an osteopathic college in London that does such a course (relatively small and relatively low-key) but the profession seems to have a fear of doctors coming in and taking over the training (this occurs both with doctors and with vets for the animal course). I would hope the profession will become more commercially aware and, while I do not believe there are thousands of doctors waiting to train as chiropractors, I think there is a small number who want this kind of training on a regular basis and who will welcome the chance to understand more about how chiropractic works, in the same way that there is a significant number who are cross-trained in osteopathy and acupuncture.

Q: What do you see as the 'sacrosanct parameters' of McTimoney chiropractic?

IP: One of the fundamental issues we all face is that the McTimoney technique has not changed since 1972. I'm absolutely sure that if John McTimoney had carried on running the College he would have changed the technique. He was an eclectic, and as new ideas appeared and his thoughts changed, he would have done whatever he felt was appropriate. That doesn't mean to say that he would have just picked up on any passing fad, but he would have been able to sense the way the market was moving, to take up new ideas and to test them out. He was a great tester of new things, and if he had lived I think by now we would be dealing with a very different technique.

Q: *At what point do you think that the technique being 'fixed' is essential to get the basics over as a teaching module?*

IP: The underpinning, the underlying philosophic view that I think is beyond dispute, is the fundamental holistic approach that everything else is based on. I firmly believe John McTimoney would have looked at all the modern developments, including the electronic equipment, and would have assessed them using the holistic fundamentals as his basis – in other words, whether it fitted in with the 'mind/body/spirit' concept, because that is where he was coming from. And if it did, and he felt it was going to aid that process, why not use it? The fundamental process for him was that the practitioner is aiding the person to heal themselves. Within our present armoury there are 37 different adjustments, but I'm sure that would have changed and there would by now be far more.

Q: *Do you think, for instance, that something like Activator technique[1] would have been approved of?*

IP: I think that's probably true. There is nothing wrong with activators, and some people are very good at using them. It is the skill of the practitioner that matters, not the piece of equipment, and that is true of a lot of pieces of equipment including your hands. There are occasions when some practitioners might be much happier using an activator, particularly those who find some aspects of the technique difficult for reasons of their own – perhaps if they suffer from arthritis – so why ignore their potential as practitioners because they can't actually do a toggle-torque-recoil, if they can find a different way of achieving the same end? If you find the right 'end' it doesn't matter (except from a purist's point of view) so long as you end up with a correct sense of purpose. If the purpose of the practitioner is correct, then it's OK.

Some people feel that the actual direct contact between their hands and the body on which they are working is paramount. There is room for plenty of different options.

One of the things that the course is looking at is moving away from the apprenticeship model (where you just learn what everybody else does and do not question) to a contextual and conceptual model where you can raise questions. The apprenticeship model may not actually be the best way of doing it, because you pick up all the bad habits as well as the good. And I think that what has been missing over the last 20 years is that some of the concepts have not been challenged. They have just been accepted as 'the tablets laid down', yet when you talk to people taught by John McTimoney, in fact he changed frequently, and didn't take a purist view of anything.

We must challenge everything in the light of current research and current experience. These are not mutually exclusive. There seems to be a reasoning around that 'if it is research, it is not necessarily pertinent, but if it's experience it's very pertinent.' That can't be right! You have got to look beyond your experience to learn. Your own experience is self-feedback within your own loop. It is subjective. What we need is a big dose of objectivity. That doesn't mean that you give up all your principles and adopt somebody else's principles. What you do is to challenge your beliefs by being open-minded about what other people are doing, and if at the end of the day you come back to what you originally believed, in a more reinforced way, that's fine. At least you are then working from the confidence of knowing that you have challenged your assumptions. If you have worked and never challenged your assumptions, that's like an act of faith, and turns your work into a religion that is unassailable. You can always hide behind 'This is what I believe in and I am not going to listen to what you are saying.' That way of thinking is not relevant to a modern profession. That is the challenge that we are going through at the moment: to let go of the past and see the new challenge without letting go of our principles.

Q: *What would you pinpoint as the main challenges of the future?*

IP: One of the identifying characteristics of an emerging profession is the setting of academic standards beyond those held by current practitioners, as a means of filtering new entrants to the profession. Nursing has done this, and now so has chiropractic. This means that practitioners who qualified in the past will have a more experiential sort of learning, but those qualifying now are going to have had a more academic training. One of the challenges for the future is how we are going to be able to cope with the different levels of training.

Q: *Is this sort of updating the purpose of Continuing Practitioner Development (CPD)?*

IP: The purpose of CPD is to have practitioners continually updating and moving forward. It brings together people who are essentially individuals, working in their own practices – giving an awareness of what others are doing, and also giving a common standard across the profession. It is very easy to become completely absorbed in your own practice and what's happening in your own world. One of the differences between an occupation and a profession is having a broader vision. Even though you've got your head down, working away, you should have the idea that you are part of a group of people who are pushing the profession forward. Your personal experience can feed into others' experience, and there is then an exchange of ideas that's invaluable. You can take up academic ideas, test them out in your practice and feed them back to the academics.

Q: *It is easier for the academic to put together a good seminar; it's much harder for the experiential practitioner to pass an experience on, yet if this doesn't happen, won't CPD become academically overloaded and thus unbalanced?*

IP: True, but there have to be ways the experiential practitioner passes back that information – perhaps through conferences and newsletters. The profession should be able to feed off itself and feed in from outside as well. There have to be loops in place to allow that to happen, because we all know of people working away by themselves, doing superb work, yet nobody outside ever gets to hear about it. I don't know of a system that monitors qualitatively as well as quantitatively; perhaps we should follow the example of the school system. It's the same old story at present. Of the people who come to conferences, 20 per cent of the profession is active, 80 per cent is not. It's not that they are not interested, they just won't participate.

The Future of McTimoney Chiropractic

Animal Chiropractic

Q: What about the field of animal chiropractic?

IP: We currently have the only externally validated course in Europe at post-graduate level. The potential for that course is huge – not only in the UK, but worldwide. I think it is the sort of course that would do well in Australia, the US and Hong Kong – places where there are people who are prepared to pay to have their animals looked after. The course has been seriously under-resourced and needs to be exploited properly. It is a very good course, giving people the opportunity to see not only where they are going, two or three years down the line, but also the result of their work very quickly under their hands. We have already attracted the osteopaths into running a parallel course, and the physiotherapists are interested in a similar course worldwide.

The new course covers all the subjects covered in a vet's training and is taught by vets, so that communication, co-operation and understanding both ways with vets are good, and the new students coming through have an underpinning knowledge of science. The course will be the basis of an MSc, which we can then develop as a PhD at such time as there is the confidence within the profession to take it on, equal to that of the veterinary sciences.

We then spoke to Dr Christina Cunliffe:

Q: What do you see is the future of McTimoney chiropractic?

CC: I agree with Ian Pearson, in that I think that it is going to be difficult for independent colleges to sustain themselves. It is essential that the McTimoney Chiropractic College (MCC) diversifies. At the moment we are a one-product business, and that is never sustainable. You have only to look at the AECC, where I believe a significant proportion of their funding comes from merchandising and other activities. I think we have to look at new revenue streams, and then it is possible and achievable for the MCC to sustain itself.

At a basic business level we can re-sell books to students, but we could also make far more use of student clinics as a revenue-generating part of the College. The important thing is how we market our franchises. I think it is going to be important to expand into Europe and lock on to US courses as well.

As far as franchising is concerned, I don't get a sense that anything is off-limits. If we choose to go that route, then we could remain independent, and this seems to be an important element for McTimoney people philosophically. Maintaining the viability of the College is crucial for the register. I also think we could market it better.

Q: In what ways?

CC: There are opportunities for approaching other universities, and getting other validations. We should develop our home market first, of course.

We have to get a foothold in a European country – perhaps Scandinavia or Holland – somewhere where there is a natural affinity with English. We need to expand into the US too. We cannot remain just UK-based, and we cannot remain isolated.

McTimoney and McTimoney-Corley

Q: Do you see there being a closer tie-up with McTimoney-Corley?

CC: I would like to think that we could come together in some way. How we do that I don't know yet, but I don't think it is sensible to remain separate in the long run. We need to know more about each other, the similarities as well as the differences. If you consider that we are all taught to common academic educational standards, McTimoney-Corley is just a slightly different practical training pathway.

Q: How do you see the development of the technique?

CC: I think it must develop, but we don't have any structures in place to monitor or feed in changes to the technique. We are initiating a research feasibility study at present, which will place the technique in space and time. It will say, 'This is how we did it in 1998–9.' Changes which practitioners develop need to be put into some sort of rigorous cycle of examination before being incorporated back into the course – it would be crucially important in how you decide which should or should not be incorporated. A lot of practitioners are keen that the McTimoney Chiropractic Association (MCA) should be guardians of the technique, but do they mean the guardians of it as it is, or guardians of its development?

Q: How will the MCA change?

CC: It has to change with the opening of the register. We should not say 'We can only afford this, so what should we do for it?' I'd prefer us to look at it the other way round –

what role do we want to play, and how do we fund it? I believe the MCA will still have an important role – but a different one. It will have a role in preserving the technique, in teaching it through the College and in supporting practitioners and the McTimoney technique. At the same time we have to be open to suggestions, but so far, discussions have tended to feed off the past and not be about new ways of thinking. People tend to get rooted in where they came from, and don't think so much about where they are going. There is a view that says the General Chiropractic Council will take over everything that the Associations do now, but the answer will have to evolve. We are not clear enough yet about the effects of opening the register, the impact of the GCC, and how *all* chiropractors will view that change.

There could also be a role for the Association down the research line. If the MCA became the developer of the technique then certainly there would be a role to foster research for the good of both practitioners and patients.

Conclusions

Observing the McTimoney scene overall, certain factors stand out. These are the machine-free approach so applicable to third-world countries, the franchise possibilities, and the future roles of both the MCA and the MCC.

The use of the hands only, in both the human and animal treatment, is specific and special to McTimoney. One of its great strengths is that it uses no X-rays or other equipment and is thus highly portable. All you need is the training, a treatment couch and a suitable patient environment, which can be set up anywhere. Because the treatment is gentle, it can also be used to treat conditions that are perhaps contra-indicated to other manipulative methods, thus providing patient choice (where there might otherwise be none).

McTimoney chiropractors do not aspire to replace doctors or vets, but to work *with* them as a complementary profession, not as an alternative one. This attitude extends into the treatment, in that practitioners work with the body, they do not impose upon it. This also makes the technique more acceptable to countries where there are more esoteric healing philosophies.

John McTimoney assembled a wonderful technique – so good that while it worked brilliantly when performed by him, it also survived him, and now works without him – the mark of a great legacy. The MCA needs to continue in the same direction. Its members need to work *on* the business, at least as much as *in* it. We need to improve efficiency as well as patient numbers; to look at selling the business (of producing chiropractors) instead of focusing only on the product (helping people heal themselves), which will happen anyway if we have more chiropractors. We need to look at how to pass on John McTimoney's message more efficiently.

If some UK areas acted as a testing ground for a franchise prototype, there is no reason why expansion into other areas of the world should not run parallel. To make such a franchise prototype does not denature the technique. The manual exists, the other aspects need to be tabulated, not as a fossilized relic to be jealously guarded against all-comers, but as a kernel that encapsulates the essence of the technique, and from which we grow and flourish.

While many chiropractors come into the profession to deal with people, not paperwork, they cannot escape paperwork altogether if they are to run an efficient business. At the same time, modern business methods are about relationships, about inspiration and imagination, about being proactive, yet listening to and learning from, the people who matter most, our patients. At all levels we need continually to ask our customers what they want from us, what they think we do well and what is not good. This information needs to be collected, collated and used as a resource to act upon.

The MCA too has customers, its practitioners. The fear that the GCC will take over everything is unjustified. It is there to safeguard the public. The MCA (in conjunction with the other three chiropractic associations, the BAAC, BCA and SCA) should be ready to defend their practitioners, to arrange group insurance and bulk merchandise, to take the lead in Continuing Practitioner Development and, last but not least, be the arbiters of what is taught as McTimoney technique (new or old).

There is a plentiful richness and cross-fertilization to be had with the other associations, and also with other alternative and complementary techniques. We are moving into a world of opportunities, for chiropractic as a whole and McTimoney chiropractic in particular. McTimoney technique can and should take its place on the world stage. It is a time of change and a time of growth, and McTimoney chiropractic will need to embrace the future wholeheartedly. This does not mean it has to compromise its philosophy or the basics of the McTimoney technique. They must not be lost, but enriched.

Appendix A

THE DIFFERENCES BETWEEN CHIROPRACTIC AND OSTEOPATHY

An often asked question is 'How does chiropractic differ from osteopathy?' Although the two disciplines developed in isolation from each other, both chiropractors and osteopaths say that more differences may be found between individual practitioners than between the two groups as a whole. They have borrowed techniques from each other.

Osteopaths treat the spine for a range of problems similar to those that confront chiropractors. Traditionally they view the body mainly as a fluid system, and to them, 'the rule of the artery is supreme'. They remove muscular inhibition of movement by soft tissue massage and then use the 'long levers' of the body to pull bones into place; for example they may release a locked joint in the middle or lower section of the spine by massaging out the muscle spasm and levering or pulling and twisting the pelvis or torso while holding the shoulders. Using the long levers gives good 'fine' control on the amount of twist and depth of adjustment, but less control on direction.

Chiropractors, in contrast, traditionally view the body as a network of nerves which control every function of the body – even the size of the arteries. They use a short-lever, high-velocity, low-amplitude thrust – that is, a short, sharp, precisely directed thrust on the joint itself to push the bones into alignment. The speed of adjustment overcomes any muscular resistance.

As to their comparative effectiveness, obviously some practitioners are more gifted manipulators than others, and as yet no comparative trials have been undertaken. Both therapies have now come under British Registration laws to ensure uniformity of basic educational and technical standards.

Appendix B

THE DIFFERENCES BETWEEN MAINSTREAM (DIVERSIFIED) TECHNIQUE AND McTIMONEY TECHNIQUE

Before explaining this in detail it is essential to understand the basic anatomy of an articulating joint. Bones are not hard and dead, but slightly springy and very much alive. A joint occurs where two adjacent bones meet and have specially designed 'articulating surfaces' covered by a very smooth substance (hyaline) to reduce friction. The joint is stabilized by ligaments and surrounded by the joint capsule, a bag of tough fibre which contains a small amount of lubricating fluid.

Because the joint capsule and ligaments stabilize the joint they also restrict the way it can move, but it is the muscles (which are highly elastic and are attached to the bones) which actually move the joint, not the ligaments (which are almost inelastic).

Movement of a joint can be active or passive. Active movement is the normal movement done by the muscles and tendons pulling on the bones either side of the joint. When the joint is moved passively by outside forces (i.e. when someone else such as the practitioner moves the patient's joint) it will be seen that there is a slightly larger range of movement possible. Passive movement uses the small amount of springy leeway available in every joint. When pushed this far, the joint will spring back to its normal active range of movement. Any gross movement beyond this can compromise the joint integrity, cause over-stretching of the ligaments and damage the capsule.

Mainstream (Diversified) Technique

The aim of a Mainstream or Diversified Technique adjustment is to increase the range of movement available in a compromised joint. The joint is taken to the end of its active range of motion, the extra, passive range is taken up by adding tension to take up the natural springiness, and the joint is then adjusted in a precise and controlled way by pushing swiftly and briefly beyond this physiological barrier into the remaining available space (known as the paraphysiological space). This gaps the joint slightly, but stops short of upsetting the integrity of the joint capsule.

This type of adjustment is frequently accompanied by a sharp 'crack'. It is thought that the sound comes from the sudden separation of the joint surfaces (cavitation) and the release of gases that were dissolved in the synovial or joint lubricating fluid, at sub-atmospheric pressure. The gap left can temporarily be seen on X-ray. The gas bubbles slowly dissolve back into the joint fluid over time, and the joint space eventually returns to its original position (which is why it is very difficult to elicit repeated cracks). However, the joint appears to retain an increased mobility in all its ranges of movement, not just in the direction of adjustment. Over-adjustment may even cause hyper-mobility.

Such a very specific type of adjustment implies a very precise differential diagnosis. Suitability of the type of adjustment (rotary or straight), including its exact line of drive and depth of adjustment, are assessed. This is why a Diversified Technique adjustment is only carried out after initial history-taking, neurological and orthopaedic tests, muscle testing and diagnostic motion palpation to determine the current position of the joint and its ability to move, in the context of a treatment plan. Often adjustments are made only after X-rays have been taken to confirm the joint's position and eliminate pathology. Records are kept according to the position of the *body* of each malpositioned vertebra and each adjustment made. This type of diagnosis lends itself well to a scientific and uantitative methodology of research, but in the process the whole-body overview and philosophical sides of chiropractic may be lost.

McTimoney Technique

In contrast, McTimoney chiropractic is a form of 'straight' or pure chiropractic (using only the hands and no other modalities such as ultrasound or X-rays) in the Vitalist tradition (*see Chapter 1*). Assessment of spinal alignment is by static palpation (feeling where the bones are without moving them). A full-body assessment is performed at every visit, and the practitioner treats 'as found' on each visit. The series of extremely fast and light adjustments have the cumulative effect of working with the body's innate healing power to find its natural position, rather than having an adjustment imposed upon it.

The main type of adjustment used over the entire spine is *toggle-torque-recoil*. The toggle is the thrust, the torque is applied during the thrust, and the recoil is the immediate removal of the practitioner's hands, allowing the patient's body to react by itself, so that the adjustment is not imposed upon it. This technique respects the body's innate knowledge of what is appropriate for it at that moment.

Such other adjustments as are used are *sprung*, employing what is known as practitioner 'follow through' so that the patient's body can find its appropriate position at or following the treatment. The paraphysiological joint space is not breached and cavitation is thus extremely rare. There is no rotary patient positioning and X-rays are not taken. Patients may be referred back to their doctor for X-rays to rule out pathology or for further tests, but these are not considered to be part of McTimoney chiropractic.

The addition of torque to an adjustment has four main benefits:

1 It is more mechanically focused and effective in depth than drive alone, and helps to open the joint space.

2 The direction of torque can be adjusted to promote a reduction in tilt and rotation of a misaligned vertebra.

3 Just as rubbing a painful spot reduces pain, a torque stimulates the faster superficial nerve fibres in the skin, which override the slower, deeper fibres that carry the sensations of pain. This means less pain is registered by the brain and the treatment is more comfortable to receive.

4 The torque effect on the skin promotes increased blood supply to the area, which aids healing.

An example of the effectiveness of whole-body treatment might be as follows:

Weak thigh muscles or pain in the thighs might suggest an upper lumbar misalignment (L1–3), and may be treated as such; however the misalignment will recur if it is due to a mechanical chain of events, as in the case of a dropped longitudinal arch in the foot causing a change in the alignment of the shin bones as they relate to the thigh bones, with subsequent poor tracking of the kneecap and pelvic misalignment; compensation for these events occurs in the most flexible part of the lumbar spine (L3). The causative correction is therefore applied to the dropped arch in the foot, not the lumbar spine, which will frequently immediately correct itself.

A whole-body treatment would discover the foot problem as a matter of course during the series of homeostatic checks and balances involved in every McTimoney treatment. Each treatment aims to return the patient's body to as good an alignment as it is able to accept that day, facilitating and respecting the patient's own innate healing ability. The aim is to work in partnership with the patient's body as it is at that time, not as part of a prefixed treatment plan over several weeks.

The Differences Between Mainstream & McTimoney Technique

Management of the patient evolves in weekly treatments depending upon response and body use in the intervening time. To this end, patients are educated in exercises and other rehabilitative measures to counteract any bad postural habits and occupational misuse. The treatment works whether the chiropractor or patient understands why it works or not.

Records are kept of all adjustments made at each treatment according to the position of the *spinous process* of the vertebra concerned. A toggle-torque-recoil adjustment has no such specificity as is found in Diversified Technique, yet it is undoubtedly remarkably effective. Qualitative rather than quantitative research methodologies are therefore far more applicable here, for example as including rather than excluding such matters as how the patient feels that day (not normally part of quantitative research methodology).

Appendix C

THE DIFFERENCES BETWEEN McTIMONEY AND McTIMONEY-CORLEY TECHNIQUES

Hugh Corley was taught by John McTimoney, but having very large hands he found he could not adjust very small areas in either humans or animals. Shelagh James-Hudson found that Corley's method also allowed her to practise chiropractic, as she was unable to extend her wrists enough to place her hands in the traditional chiropractic hand position. Together they developed a technique and formed the McTimoney-Corley School, now called The Oxford College of Chiropractic.

The differences between McTimoney and McTimoney-Corley techniques are small but significant. They are found in:

1 the method of palpation and adjustment

2 the order of treatment

3 the amount of mobilization techniques

4 the shape of the adjusting table.

Method of Palpation and Adjustment

The main finger used to feel the placement of bones – the palpation finger – in McTimoney-Corley technique is the index rather than the middle finger. When palpating the spine, the index fingers rest either side of the spinous process of each vertebra and both the middle and ring fingers trail with the index finger. They pick up information about the intrinsic and local musculature of the spine as well as the transverse processes of each vertebra.

To adjust a misaligned vertebra using the McTimoney-Corley technique, rather than doing a toggle-recoil on the transverse process of that vertebra, the middle and possibly the ring fingers are placed at right angles to the spine, on the side of the spinous process of the misaligned vertebra. The other hand is placed across these fingers and provides the impetus for a flick across the spine, which mobilizes both the bone and the surrounding tissues. The vertebra then responds with a reflex-recoil to find a better position.

When treating babies, children and small animals, the reflex-recoil adjustment is used. The pisiform adjustment (normally used by McTimoney practitioners) is used only for large animals.

The Order of Treatment

While the general method of assessment is the same, the atlas, all cranial adjustments and all arm, wrist and hand adjustments are carried out with the patient in the seated position. These are completed before the patient goes to lie supine (face up) on the table for pelvic adjustments. The side-lying ischial (sitting bone) adjustments follow the prone (face-down) adjustments instead of preceding them.

The Amount of Mobilization Techniques

The general McTimoney-Corley protocol employs more mobilization techniques than the McTimoney protocol. With the patient supine, the leg mobilizations include versions of two orthopaedic tests (McMurray's and Fabère). The pelvic adjustments are done as part of a rolling mobilization; the sacro-iliac joint (between the back of the pelvis and sacrum) is mobilized and the quadratus lumborum muscles are stretched.

Prone adjustments include mobilization of all spinous processes of the thoracic and lumbar vertebrae, prior to revisiting those vertebrae needing adjustment. Side-lying treatment includes mobilization of the femoral head (top of the thigh bone) in the acetabulum (hip joint).

The patient is asked to walk about the treatment room briefly, before the final seated check, which may include neck stretches and shoulder-blade mobilization.

The Differences Between McTimoney & McTimoney-Corley Techniques

The Shape of the Adjusting Table

The table most commonly used by McTimoney chiropractors is narrower at the head-end to allow close proximity for neck adjustments. McTimoney equipment includes an adjustable stool or headpiece for the patient's head, while McTimoney-Corley technique originally began by treating patients on the floor (because then the practitioner could stand over the patient and work centrally). Now a fixed, square-ended or slightly tapered table is used.

It must be emphasized that both McTimoney and McTimoney-Corley techniques always do a whole-body assessment and treatment at every visit. Both are done in the same spirit and philosophy, based on a partnership with the patient's body to help it heal itself, by working with and facilitating its innate healing ability. Nothing is imposed. In both techniques, all mobilization is done within the normal range of movement and no adjustment enters the paraphysiological space (*see Appendix B*).

REFERENCES

Chapter 1

1. See Appendix A for a comparison between osteopathy and chiropractic.
2. Sections of the protruding parts of each vertebra, to which muscles are attached.
3. A word used since the 17th century, and the subject of a doctoral thesis by Johan Heinrich Hieronymi in 1746.
4. Russell W. Gibbons, in Scott Haldemann (ed), *Modern Developments in the Principles and Practice of Chiropractic* (New York, 1979).
5. op cit.

Chapter 2

1. From an account written by John McTimoney in the late 1960s.

Chapter 5

1. Mannheim, J., *Modern Maturity* June/July 1989: page 76.
2. Clinical Standards Advisory Group Backpain Report, HMSO 1994.
3. 'Acute low back problems in adults', Clinical Practice Guide no. 14 (US Dept of Health and Human Services; Public Health Service Agency for Health Care Policy and Research, Rockville, Maryland, Dec. 1994).
4. Braaf, M. and Rosner S., 'Trauma of the cervical spine as cause of chronic headache', *Trauma* 15 (1975): pages 441–6.
5. Radler, M., 'Dysmenorrhea', *The American Chiropractor* March/April 1984.

Chapter 6

1. Winspur, I., FRCS FACS (1995).

Chapter 7

1. Gutman, G., 'Blocked Atlantal Nerve Syndrome in Babies and Infants', *Manuelle Medizin* 25 (1987): pages 5–10.

Chapter 9

1. An activator is a small modified hand-held dental hammer. The light spring loading is adjustable, the hammer head is the size of a 1-penny piece. Adjustments feel like a normal toggle-recoil but without the torque.

BIBLIOGRAPHY AND FURTHER READING

1997 Client Survey Results (Eynsham: MCA, 1997)

Andrews, Elizabeth. *Muscle Management* (Thorsons, 1991)

—. *Healthy Practice for Musicians* (Rhinegold, 1997)

Bach, Marcus. *The Chiropractic Story* (Georgia: Si-Nel Publishing, 1986)

Braaf, M and Rosner, S. 'Trauma of the cervical spine as cause of chronic headache', *Trauma* 15 (1975): pages 441–6.

British Medical Association. *Alternative Therapy* (BMA, 1986)

—. *Complementary Medicine* (BMA, 1993)

Carrington, M. 'The attitudes of GPs towards communication with manipulative practitioners' (unpublished paper, March 1998)

Cartlidge, Susan, BA, MC, MMCA. *Healthy Backs – Healthy Children* (report to Parliamentary Sub-Committee, MCA, Eynsham, 1996)

Chiropractic Registration Steering Group Ltd. *Report of a Working Party on Current Parameters for Safe and Competent Practice in Chiropractic* (CRSG, Braintree, 1995)

Clinical Guidelines for the Management of Acute Low Back Pain (Royal College of General Practitioners, London, 1998)

Clinical Standards Advisory Group. *Back Pain Report* (HMSO, 1994)

Commission of Inquiry into Chiropractic, *Chiropractic in New Zealand* (Hasselburg [Government Printer], Wellington, 1979)

Courtenay, Anthea. *Chiropractic for Everyone, your spine and your health* (Penguin, 1987)

Haldemann, Scott (ed). *Modern Developments in the Principles and Practice of Chiropractic* (NY: Appleton-Century-Crofts, 1980)

Harding, Stanley. *McTimoney Chiropractic, the first 25 years* (McTimoney Chiropractic Association, 1997)

Inglis, Brian. *Fringe Medicine* (Faber & Faber, 1964)

—. *Natural Medicine* (Fontana/Collins, 1979/80)

Manga, P et al. *The Effectiveness and Cost-effectiveness of Chiropractic Management of Low-back Pain* (University of Ottawa: Pran Manga and Associates, 1993)

Palmer, D D. *The Chiropractor* (LA: 1914; republished by Health Research, California, 1970)

Palmer, David D, BS, DC. *Three Generations: A Brief History of Chiropractic* (Davenport, IA: Palmer College of Chiropractic, 1967)

Radler, M. 'Dysmenorrhea', *The American Chiropractor* March/April 1984

Winspur, I. 'The professional musician and the hand surgeon', *Performing Arts Medicine News* 3.3

USEFUL ADDRESSES

McTimoney Chiropractic
  Association
21 High Street
Eynsham
Oxford OX8 1HE
Tel: 01865 880974
Fax: 01865 880975

McTimoney Chiropractic College
The Clock House
22–26 Ock Street
Abingdon
Oxon OX14 5SH
Tel: 01235 523336
Fax: 01235 523255

National Back Pain Association
16 Elmtree Road
Teddington
Middlesex TW11 8ST
Tel: 0181 977-5474
Fax: 0181 943-5318

INDEX

195